1 MONTH OF
FREE
READING

at

www.ForgottenBooks.com

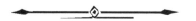

By purchasing this book you are eligible for one month membership to ForgottenBooks.com, giving you unlimited access to our entire collection of over 700,000 titles via our web site and mobile apps.

To claim your free month visit:
www.forgottenbooks.com/free251484

ISBN 978-0-260-84559-7
PIBN 10251484

The All-England Series

GYMNASTICS

BY
A. F. JENKIN.

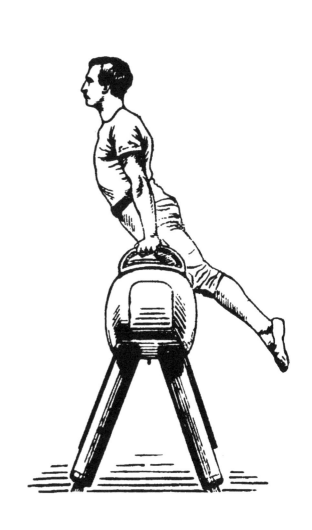

F. H. AYRES,

MANUFACTURER OF

ALL SPORTS & GAMES,

111, Aldersgate Street, London.

GYMNASTIC APPARATUS,

HORIZONTAL BARS.

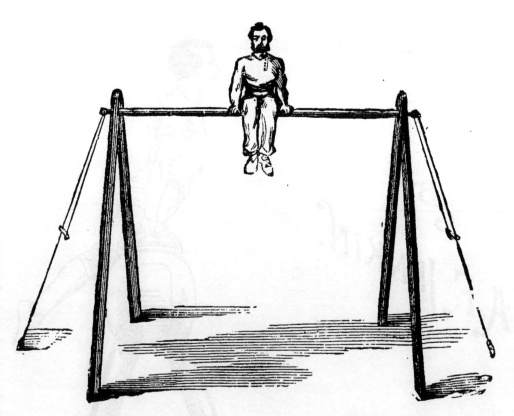

ILLUSTRATED CATALOGUES ON APPLICATION.

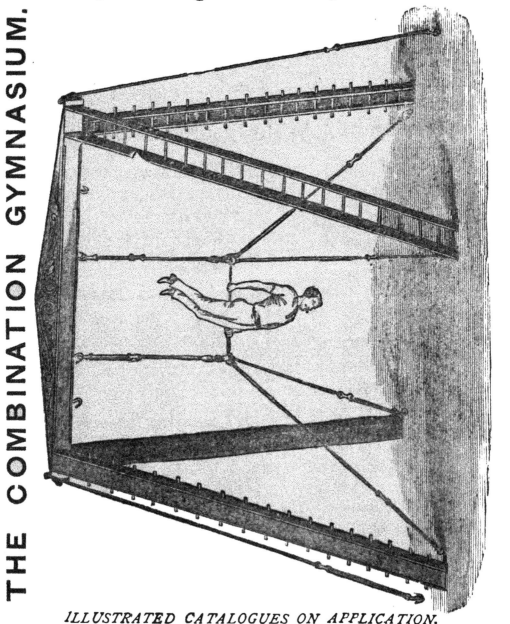

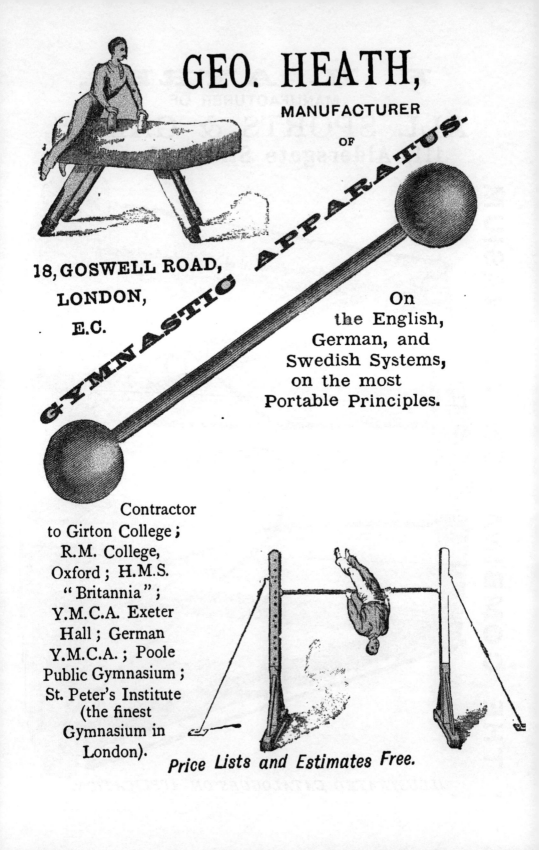

GEO. HEATH,

MANUFACTURER

OF

GYMNASTIC APPARATUS.

18, GOSWELL ROAD,
LONDON,
E.C.

On
the English,
German, and
Swedish Systems,
on the most
Portable Principles.

Contractor
to Girton College;
R.M. College,
Oxford; H.M.S.
"Britannia";
Y.M.C.A. Exeter
Hall; German
Y.M.C.A.; Poole
Public Gymnasium;
St. Peter's Institute
(the finest
Gymnasium in
London).

Price Lists and Estimates Free.

The Club Series

OF CARD AND TABLE GAMES.

Small 8vo, cloth, price 1s. each.

WHIST. By Dr. William Pole, F.R.S., author of "The Philosophy of Whist," etc.

SOLO WHIST. By Robert F. Green, editor of "Chess."

BILLIARDS. The Art of Practical Billiards for Amateurs ; with chapters on POOL, PYRAMIDS, and SNOOKER. By Major-General A. W. Drayson, F.R.A.S., author of "Practical Whist." With a Preface by W. J. Peall. *With Illustrations.*

CHESS. By Robert F. Green, editor of the "British Chess Magazine." *With Illustrations.*

CHESS PROBLEMS. A Collection of Two-Move Problems. By B. G. LAWS.

DRAUGHTS and BACKGAMMON. By "Berkeley." *With Illustrations.*

REVERSI and GO BANG. By "Berkeley." *With Illustrations.*

DOMINOES and SOLITAIRE. By "Berkeley." *With Illustrations.*

BÉZIQUE and CRIBBAGE. By "Berkeley."

ÉCARTÉ and EUCHRE. By "Berkeley."

PIQUET. By "Berkeley."

ROUND GAMES, including Poker, Loo, Vingt-et-un, Napoleon, Newmarket, Rouge et Noir, Pope Joan, Speculation, etc., etc.

Preparing.

LONDON : G. BELL & SONS.

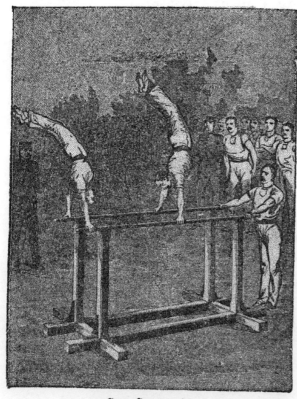

GYMNASTICS.

A. F. JENKIN.

THE ALL-ENGLAND SERIES.

Small 8vo, cloth, price 1s. each.

CRICKET. By the HON. AND REV. E. LYTTELTON.

LAWN TENNIS. By H. W. W. WILBERFORCE, Sec. A.E.L.T.C.

TENNIS, RACKETS, and FIVES. By JULIAN MAR-SHALL, MAJOR SPENS, and REV. J. ARNAN TAIT.

GOLF. By W. T. LINSKILL, Cam. Univ. Golf Club.

HOCKEY. By F. S. CRESWELL. [*In paper cover*, 6d.]

ROWING AND SCULLING. By W. B. WOODGATE, Diamond Sculls.

SAILING. By E. F. KNIGHT, Author of " The Cruise of the 'Falcon,'" &c. [*Double volume*, 2s.]

SWIMMING. By M. and J. R. COBBETT.

BOXING. By R. G. ALLANSON-WINN, Winner of Middle and Heavy Weights, Cambridge, 1876-8.

WRESTLING. By WALTER ARMSTRONG, Author of " Wrestliana."

FENCING. By H. A. COLMORE DUNN, Inns of Court School of Arms.

SINGLESTICK AND SWORD EXERCISE. By R. G. ALLANSON-WINN and C. PHILLIPPS-WOLLEY.

FOOTBALL—RUGBY GAME. By HARRY VASSALL.

FOOTBALL — ASSOCIATION GAME. By C. W. ALCOCK.

SKATING. By DOUGLAS ADAMS, London Skating Club. With numerous Illustrations. [*Double volume*, 2s.]

CYCLING. By H. H. GRIFFIN, L.A.C., N.C.U., C.T.C.

ATHLETICS. By H. H. GRIFFIN, L.A.C.

GYMNASTICS. By A. F. JENKIN, German Gymnastic Society, etc. [*Double volume*, 2s.]

CLUBS. By G. T. B. COBBETT and A. F. JENKIN.
Preparing.

DUMB-BELLS. *Preparing.*

ROUNDERS, BASEBALL, BOWLS, QUOITS, etc. By J. M. WALKER. *Preparing.*

RIDING. By W. A. KERR, V.C. *Preparing.*

DRIVING. _____ *Preparing.*

LONDON: GEORGE BELL & SONS.

GYMNASTICS.

BY

A. F. JENKIN,

GERMAN GYMNASTIC SOCIETY, AND INNS OF COURT SCHOOL OF
ARMS, WINNER OF THE GERMAN GYMNASTIC SOCIETY'S
CHALLENGE CUP, 1887-8-9.

WITH ILLUSTRATIONS.

LONDON: GEORGE BELL & SONS, YORK STREET,
COVENT GARDEN.

1890.

PREFACE.

THE following pages are devoted to the discussion of gymnastics from the point of view of a learner who desires to become a fine gymnast. No attempt has been made to deal with the medical aspect of the subject, nor has space been given to the description of abnormal feats of strength and dexterity. My main object has been to describe as great a variety of exercises as possible, and to describe them in such a way that the reader, even though he has no previous knowledge of the subject, may be able to set about learning them with a clear idea of what he should try to do.

The illustrations, with the exception of a few diagrams, are reproduced from instantaneous photographs taken by Mr. George Mitchell, of Lewisham. In taking these no recourse was had to artificial supports; in every instance the actual exercise illustrated was done and photographed.

Thanks are due from me to Mr. J. W. Macqueen and to other friends for valuable assistance.

A. F. JENKIN.

7, CROWN OFFICE ROW, TEMPLE,
1890.

CONTENTS.

GYMNASTICS.

CHAPTER I.

INTRODUCTION.

§ 1. Introductory—§§ 2–7. Style—§ 8. Arrangement of Chapters—§§ 9–17. Nomenclature.

§ 1. In the present chapter it is my intention, first, to give some general hints as to the style in which exercises should be done and as to the way in which a correct style may be acquired; and, secondly, to explain the arrangement adopted and the system of nomenclature employed in the subsequent chapters.

The suggestions as to style contained in the next few paragraphs are of the greatest importance; for, in gymnastics, to parody a well-known saying, there are three essentials—the first is style, the second is style, and the third is style. Strength you will acquire naturally, if you do plenty of work, and dexterity you will acquire unconsciously with practice; but style you can only acquire by constant attention, and then only if you have a clear idea of what to aim at.

The general explanations as to nomenclature contained in §§ 10–13 are essential to the understanding of the subsequent chapters. The remaining paragraphs are devoted

B

to the discussion of certain difficulties connected with nomenclature, and are, I fear, somewhat abstruse; they are, however, addressed to practised gymnasts only, and may be omitted by beginners.

STYLE.

§ 2. *Carriage of the Head.* As a rule, whenever the main portion of the body is erect, the head should be carried erect. You will find that the position of the head depends upon the direction in which you are looking. If you look up, your head will be erect; if you look down, you will stoop. Therefore, unless there is some special reason against it, whenever your position is in the main upright, you should look at a point rather above the level of your eyes. It is possible to keep the eyes up while stooping by poking the chin forward; but, if you keep the chin well pressed back, and the eyes fixed on a point above their own level, your head is almost certain to be in a correct position. In order to acquire a correct carriage of the head you must learn to avoid looking at the apparatus on which you are working. At first this requires some resolution, especially if you have to shift your grasp, but you will soon learn to know instinctively where the apparatus is without looking at it.

§ 3. *Carriage of the Legs and Feet.* As a rule you should keep the legs perfectly straight, with the toes as much pointed as possible. You cannot keep the legs in this position without bracing the muscles; your legs will not hang straight, you must hold them straight; stretch them straight, in fact. Again, as a rule, you should keep the legs together so that they are in contact at the knee, the ankle, and at the ball of the foot. Even the most practised gymnasts in doing an unwonted exercise cannot be sure for themselves that their legs have not bent or separated, and beginners often double the knees till the feet nearly touch the thighs, and separate the legs wide, quite unconsciously.

§ 4. *Beginning Exercises—Position of "Attention."* In beginning an exercise, in which the movement proper is begun from a standing position, you should walk straight up to the apparatus, stand for an instant with the heels together, the toes turned slightly out, the head and body erect, and the arms by the sides, and then, without hesitation, spring or grasp the apparatus as the case may be. In beginning exercises which are done after running up to the apparatus, you should stand for an instant at a suitable distance from the apparatus in the position described above, and then, without hesitation, walk two or three paces forwards, so as to get into your stride, and then begin to run without any shuffling of the feet or changing step. Although there is little difficulty in beginning exercises properly, your exercises will gain greatly in finish if you attend to the point. The standing position described above is called the position of "attention."

§ 5. *Leaving the Apparatus.* In alighting from an apparatus, you should, just before you reach the ground, bend the knees slightly, separate them, and turn the toes out, keeping the muscles of the legs braced, and the eyes fixed on a point slightly above their own level. Then pitch on the toes, let the knees bend further, and then straighten the knees and come to the position of "attention" without shifting the feet. As you alight, the arms, unless you retain hold of the apparatus, should be kept straight, and hang outside the knees. If you are alighting from a considerable height, you should hold the arms from your sides, at right angles to the body, and let the knees bend till the heels almost touch the thighs; but in alighting from a moderate height, the knees should not bend so much, and the arms should be held only just clear of the knees.

The method described above is the only safe way of alighting from any considerable height; if you pitch on your heels, or fail to bend the knees, you may seriously jar the back; if you do not separate the knees, you may easily sprain, or even dislocate them, and you may hit your jaw badly on your knee; if the arms are not kept outside the knees, you may hit the forearm a bad blow across the knee; and, if you do not keep the eyes off the ground, your head will come forward with a jerk as you alight, which may be attended with very serious consequences. Even in alighting from quite a moderate height, you may get hurt if you are not in a proper position, and I think that more than half the sprained knees and ankles which occur in a gymnasium are due to alighting in a wrong position.

If, after alighting, you fall backwards, do not put out your hands to save yourself; bring your hands forward, raise your shoulders, bring your head into your chest and roll over, and you will not hurt yourself; if you put out your hands you may easily sprain or break the wrists.

It is of the utmost importance to learn to alight properly; in the first place for safety's sake, and, secondly, because nothing detracts more from the appearance of an exercise than alighting in a clumsy manner. The proper method of alighting can, however, only be acquired by assiduous practice. You should make it a rule never, by any chance, to alight carelessly.

§ 6. *General Style.* Exercises should, as a rule, be done with an even and continuous movement without any jerk, pause, or hurry, so that the whole exercise has a cadenced appearance. If, however, a pause is introduced in the course of an exercise, you should make a definite pause, remaining absolutely motionless for, at least, sufficient time to show that the pause is intentional; again, if an abrupt movement is introduced, that movement should, as a rule, be made as suddenly and decisively as possible. In doing slow exercises you must not hurry the difficult parts in order to get them over, nor the easy parts because they are not worth wasting time about. Provided that your movement is perfectly continuous and even, the slower you do slow exercises the better.

§ 7. *Acquisition of a Correct Style.* If you have a good instructor, it is comparatively easy to acquire a correct style, but you will have constantly to ask him whether your exercises are properly done or he may think that you know of defects of which you are perfectly unconscious, and may accordingly fail to mention them. If you have no instructor, get some one to look on; consider where you are likely to make mistakes, and direct the onlooker's attention to that particular point; explain what you are going to do, and ask him to tell you whether at a particular moment your knees are straight, or your back perfectly hollow, or your body horizontal, or whatever the particular point you want to know about may be. It is no use asking a man who does not know much about gymnastics whether your exercise, generally speaking, is well done or not; he does not know what points to attend to. Finally, remember that there is no such thing as perfection in gymnastics; however well you may do an exercise, there is always a possibility of doing it better still, and this is true even of the simplest and easiest movements.

ARRANGEMENT OF CHAPTERS.

§ 8. Each of the three principal instruments, the horse, the horizontal bar, and the parallel bars, I shall deal with in a separate chapter, describing first the leading positions on the instrument, and then the various exercises. These exercises will be divided into groups according to the nature of the movements made, and not according to their comparative difficulty.

In discussing the simpler movements I shall, as a rule, first describe a complete exercise introducing the movement in question, and then make such general remarks about the movement as may seem necessary. In discussing more complicated movements, on the other hand, I shall, as a rule, begin by a general account of a group of exercises, and then give particular examples. These examples have generally been made long and difficult in order to introduce as great a variety of movements as possible; but, for actual practice at first, you will of course find it easy to simplify them. Many exercises are unsymmetrical, that is to say, they may be done either right or left. These will be, for the sake of brevity, described to the one side only, leaving it to you to reverse them; but it is of the greatest importance to be able to do all such exercises indifferently right or left.

NOMENCLATURE.

§ 9. At the present time there is, in this country, no generally recognized system of nomenclature for the description of gymnastic exercises, and the want of some such system has been a very serious obstacle to the spread of this branch of athletics. In writing the present work, one of my main objects has been, if possible, to supply this want.

The system of nomenclature at present obtaining with the German Gymnastic Society and other leading gymnastic clubs in London, and adopted by the Amateur Gymnastic Association, is that employed by Knofe and Macqueen in their translation of Püritz' " Merkbüchlein für Vortürner," and my endeavour has been, while conforming as far as possible to that system, to place it upon a basis of accurate definitions, and to extend it to the description of the more complicated exercises. The difficulties of this undertaking have been very great, and I am conscious that, in striving after accuracy, I have at times been guilty of pedantry, and, on the other hand, that, in an effort to conform to the existing system, I have at times sacrificed simplicity and uniformity.

I have, however, had the pleasure of submitting the system employed in this book to the Committee of the Amateur Gymnastic Association, and they, after making many valuable suggestions, which I have adopted, passed a unanimous resolution expressing approval of the system. I am therefore encouraged to hope that I may to some extent attain my object, and that the present work may be instrumental in spreading the use of a uniform and established system of nomenclature in this country.

§ 10. The remaining paragraphs of the present chapter are devoted to general explanations as to the method in which movements involving a rotation are described; but, as has been already stated, it is unnecessary for a beginner to read further than to the end of § 13. Before passing on, however, I should point out that throughout the book certain common expressions, such as " right " and " left," " forwards " and " backwards," " in front of " and " behind," are used in accordance with the definitions given from time to time, and that it will be impossible for the reader to follow the descriptions of the various exercises unless he bears these definitions in mind.

§ 11. *Turns.* The meaning of the expressions "turn to the right" and "turn to the left" must be clearly understood. Imagine that you are standing on the face of a clock at the centre, and that you turn with the hands; you turn to the right; if you turn in the opposite direction, you turn to the left. Now suppose you are not upright, but in some other position; imagine that your legs are in a straight line with the body, with the feet against the face of a clock; then, if you turn with the hands, you turn to the right; if in the opposite direction, you turn to the left. For example, if you are lying down on your back and roll over on to your right side, you turn to the right. Again, if you are lying down on your face and roll over on to your right side, you turn to the left.

§ 12. *Turn of Limbs.* The expressions "turn to the right" and "turn to the left" are used not only with reference to the body, but also with reference to the limbs. For example, if you take a watch up in one hand between the fingers and thumb, with the face to the palm of the hand, as in the sketch (Fig. 1),

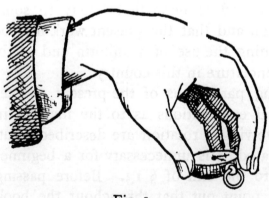

Fig. 1.

and place the hand in any position, and turn the watch in the direction in which the hands move, you turn the hand to the right; if you turn the watch in the opposite direction, you turn the hand to the left. Again, if you turn the right foot out, you turn the foot to the right; if you turn the left foot out, you turn the foot to the left. Again, if you turn the head in the direction it would move, if you held the neck stiff and made a turn to the right with the body, you turn the head to the right; if you turn the head the other way, you turn the head to the left.

§ 13. *Extent of Turn.* If you turn through four right angles, or, in other words, through a whole circle, coming again to your original position, you make a complete turn; and if you turn through any portion of four right angles, the extent of your turn is denoted with reference to a complete turn : thus a turn through one right angle is a quarter turn; so that "quarter right turn" in gymnastic language is the same thing as "right turn" in military language. Again, "half left turn" is the same thing as a "left about turn" in military language.

In a similar manner, if you turn a limb through one right angle, that limb makes a quarter turn; if through two right angles, a half turn, and so on.

§ 14. The word "turn" in gymnastic language, used with reference to the body, is confined in meaning to a rotation about an axis parallel to the backbone. You often, of course, in doing exercises perform a rotation about axes in other directions; for example, in movements in the course of which you turn head over heels, such as circles on the horizontal bar, you perform a rotation about an axis parallel to the straight line joining the points of the shoulders; but such a rotation is not called a turn.

A rotation about the last mentioned axis is denoted by the words "swing," "circle," "roll," or "somersault," and the rotations in the two directions are distinguished by the use of the words "forwards" and "backwards," or "front" and "back." In all forward or front circles, rolls, or somersaults, the rotation is with the hands of a clock placed on your left with the face towards you; in backward circles, rolls, or somersaults, the rotation is against the hands of a clock so placed. In forward swings, however, the rotation is in the same direction as in backward circles, rolls, or somersaults; and in backward swings the rotation is in the same direction as in forward circles, rolls, or somersaults.

Again, you may perform a rotation about an axis perpendicular both to the backbone and to the straight line joining the shoulders, which axis may be called for the moment the "cross axis;" as, for example, in a movement like that made in raising the body above the instrument in a flank vault, or in moving from a double elbow lever between the parallel bars to a right elbow lever. Unfortunately, no word appropriate to a rotation about the cross axis is in use at present, and the words "turn" and "swing" are often used for such movements.

§ 15. It should be pointed out that by performing a rotation about one axis, and then a rotation about another, you may reach a position which you could also reach by performing a rotation about a third axis. For example, if from a vertical position you swing to a horizontal position, and then carry the body round with a rotation about the "cross axis" through a right angle, and then drop again with a swing to a vertical position, you will find yourself in the same position as if you had done a quarter turn, that is to say, a rotation about the axis parallel to the backbone. A rotation may also, of course, be made about an axis which is not in any one of the three directions above spoken of, but it is often impossible to describe such a movement with perfect accuracy in a reasonable space, and accordingly it is necessary to be content with an approximate description of the movement, describing it as if consisting in a rotation about one of the three principal axes followed by a rotation about another.

As an example of what is meant, you may consider a front vault over the horse. You might describe this movement approximately in two ways: (1) throw the legs up to the left with a rotation about the cross axis, then do a quarter right turn, and then drop the legs with a swing; (2) swing the legs up to a free front lever, then carry the legs to the left with rotation about the cross axis, and then drop them. Now, in point of fact, in doing a front vault you really make an intermediate movement; but it would be impossible in any reasonable space to describe exactly the movement made, and accordingly you must choose that one of the two approximate descriptions suggested, which you consider most nearly accurate.

§ 16. It may be advisable to point out that it is at first by no means easy to see which way you should turn to do a right turn when in a vertical position with the legs above the head, for example, in a handstand. If you are in a handstand on the parallel bars, and turn to a handstand on the left bar, placing the right hand in front of the left, so that the thumbs of the two hands are next each other, you have done a quarter *right* turn. This seems surprising at first, but a little thought will convince you that it is so.

§ 17. If you have difficulty in understanding the last few paragraphs, I should advise you to cut a rough figure of a man out of a piece of paper, and mark his face and back, and his right and left arms and legs, then draw an arrow across his chest with the point towards his right shoulder, and then remember that if he is turning so that the arrow is moving in the direction in which it is pointing, he is turning to the right, and you will easily convince yourself by experiment that the statements in these paragraphs are accurate.

CHAPTER II.

THE HORSE.

PART I.—*EXERCISES ON HORSE PLACED SIDEWAYS WITH POMMELS.*

120, 121. Thief Jumps—§§ 122–133. Miscellaneous Exercises, Wolf Vaults, Fencing Vaults, Handstands, Elbow Levers, Examples of Combined Exercises.

APPARATUS AND GENERAL DEFINITIONS.

§ 18. A rough sketch of the horse is given in Fig. 2; the total length of the horse should be about 6 ft.; the

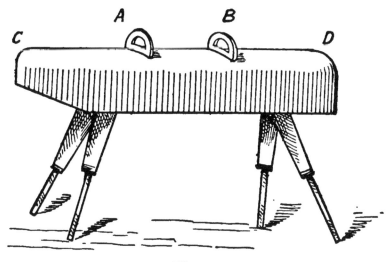

Fig. 2.

distance between the pommels, measured from centre to centre, about 17½ in.; the height of the pommels at the centre about 4¾ in. The pommels should be hollow, like hoops, and the solid part should be about 1½ in. in diameter; Fig. 3 shows roughly a cross section of the horse through one pommel. The horse should be capable of being raised and lowered, and the pommels should be removable. A small spring-

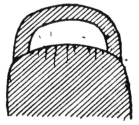

Fig. 3.

board is generally used with the horse; this should be about 3 ft. long, and about 4 in. high at the higher end.

The horse should, as a rule, be placed at about the height of the breast, reckoning from the top of the spring-board to the top of the horse itself, not to the highest point of the pommels. It is advisable to avoid practising on a horse lower than this, as it tends to produce a bad style; if the horse is placed at a greater height, on the other hand, it merely makes exercises from the ground a little more difficult.

§ 19. *Names of Various Parts of Horse.* The portion of the horse outside the pommels at the one end (C in Fig. 2) is called the neck; the portion between the pommels is called the saddle; the portion outside the pommels at the other end (D in Fig. 2) is called the croup. The pommel next the neck (A in Fig. 2) is called the neck pommel; the other, (B in Fig. 2) the croup pommel. The side of the horse on the left, looking from the croup towards the neck, is called the "near side," the other side of the horse the "off side."

The spring-board is generally placed either on the near side of the horse, or at one end of the horse close to the croup. When the spring-board is on the near side of the horse, the horse is said to be placed "sideways;" when the spring-board is placed at the end of the horse close to the croup, the horse is said to be placed "lengthways." Of course exercises may be devised with the spring-board placed obliquely to the horse. Throughout the first part of the present chapter (as far as § 133) the pommels are supposed to be on the horse, and the horse is supposed to be placed sideways.

§ 20. *Meaning of " Parallel to Horse," " At Right Angles to Horse."* The expression "parallel to the horse" means parallel to the length of the horse; and the expression "at right angles to the horse" means at right angles to the length of the horse.

POSITIONS.

§ 21. *General Rules.* So far as nothing to the contrary appears either expressly or by implication in the description of any position on the horse in which the shoulders are parallel to the horse, it is assumed—

(i.) That your body is over or opposite the saddle.

(ii.) That you are facing the off side of the horse.

§ 22. *Seats.* The principal seats on the horse are—

(i.) *The Riding Seat.* In this position you sit astride the horse, as if you were riding a real horse, but with your legs straight.

(ii.) *The Side Riding Seat.* From the riding seat turn through a quarter turn to the right, bringing the shoulders and hips parallel to the horse, at the same time turning the right leg out and the left leg in, so that the horse is grasped between the front of the left thigh and the back of the right thigh ; you are then in the "side riding seat" with the right leg forward. If you turn in the same manner from the riding seat to the left, you come to the side riding seat with the left leg forward. In the side riding seat, you must keep the weight well over the centre of the horse, so that the back is considerably hollowed.

(iii.) *The Side Seat.* In this position you sit on the horse as you would on a chair; but you should keep the legs straight, and not bend much at the waist.

(iv.) *The Cross Seat.* In this position you sit with the shoulders at right angles to the horse, and both legs on the same side of it. You may come to a cross seat with the legs in various positions; in the absence of directions to the contrary, you should sit fairly on the seat with the legs straight and nearly horizontal, and with the hips not quite at right angles to the horse, but turned somewhat towards the side of the horse on which the legs are. You may also come to a cross seat with the knee of the leg nearest the horse bent so that the back of the thigh rests on the horse, and with the other leg hanging straight down; this position is called the cross seat with one knee bent; it is almost exactly like a seat in a side saddle on a real horse. You may also come to a cross seat with the hips completely at right angles to the horse, and with the outside of one thigh in contact with the horse; this position is called the cross seat on the outside of one thigh; it is almost impossible to retain, without grasping the horse to steady yourself.

§ 23. *Rests.* Positions on the horse in which you are wholly or mainly supported on the arms, with the weight below the shoulders, are called rests. The following are the principal rests—

(i.) *The Front Rest.* In the front rest the weight is supported partly on the arms and partly on the front of the thighs. The arms should be straight, the back hollow, and the shoulders parallel to the horse. You should let the front of the thighs rest lightly against the horse, but support almost the whole weight on the arms.

(ii.) *The Back Rest.* In the back rest the weight is supported partly on the arms and partly on the back of the thighs. The arms should be straight, and the shoulders parallel to the horse. You should let the back of the thighs rest lightly against the horse, but support almost the whole weight on the arms. If you intend to pause in the back rest, the back should be hollow; but before beginning exercises from the back rest it is generally necessary to bend very slightly at the waist.

(iii.) *The Side Riding Rest.* In this position you support most of the weight on the arms, with the legs astride the horse between the arms; the arms should be straight, the back hollow, and the shoulders parallel to the horse. If you come to a side riding seat on the saddle, grasp the pommels, and support most of the weight on the arms, you reach a side riding rest on the saddle. You may in a side riding rest keep both legs in contact with the horse, or only one, raising the other clear of it; you may also raise both legs clear of the horse, and support the whole weight on the arms; but in that case the position is called a "free side riding rest."

You may come to a front rest, back rest, or riding rest, on the saddle, neck, or croup, and in each case you may place the hands in various positions. In a rest on the saddle, unless the contrary appears, you should grasp both pommels in the centre, with the back of the right hard to the right, and the back of the left hand to the left. The front rest in the saddle is shown in Fig. 4. The back rest in the saddle, with the waist slightly bent, ready to begin exercises, is shown in Fig. 5.

§ 24. *Free Rests.* The word "free," in the description of a rest, means that the legs are not to touch the horse, and that the whole weight is to be supported on the arms. The free front rest you may reach from the front rest by carrying the legs a few inches to the rear; the free back rest you may reach from the back rest by carrying the legs a few inches forward; and the free side riding rest you may, as has already been mentioned, reach from the riding rest by straddling the legs a little wider, and raising them from the horse. The free front rest is a position which cannot be retained for any appreciable time, but it is of constant occurrence in the course of exercises.

§ 25. *The Half Lever.* From the back rest, bend at the waist and raise the legs until they are horizontal, supporting

C

the whole weight on the hands; the position you then reach

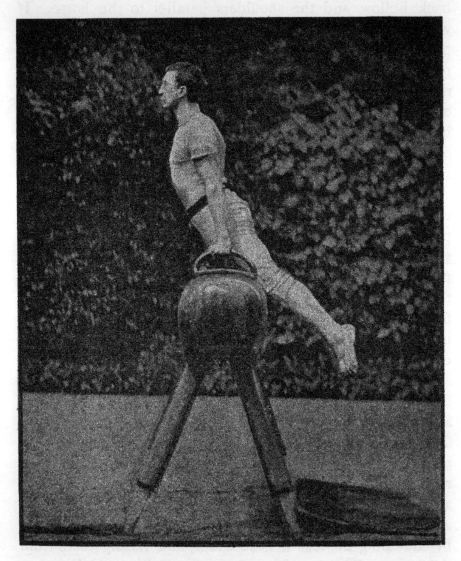

Fig. 4.—FRONT REST.

is called the "half lever." Fig. 18 shows this position on
the parallel bars.

COMMENCEMENT OF EXERCISES.

§ 26. Many exercises on the horse are begun with a run,

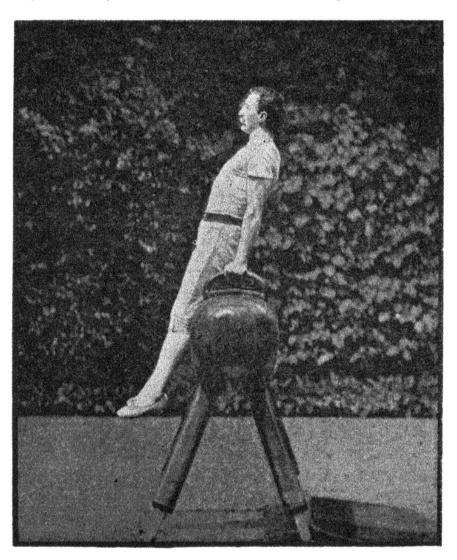

Fig. 5.—BACK REST.

and this method of beginning an exercise requires explanation. Stand facing the horse about ten yards from it, run

towards the horse, spring from one foot and alight on both
feet on the spring-board, then spring from both feet, grasping
the horse at the same moment. The expression, "with a
run," at the beginning of the description of an exercise,
means that the exercise is to be begun in this manner.
There are exercises which are begun by running and springing from the spring-board from one foot, or by springing
without grasping the horse; but, in describing these exercises, the expression " with a run " is not used.

VAULTS.

§ 27. *With a Run, Flank Vault Left over Saddle.* Run,
grasp the pommels, and spring, as described in § 26, let go
with the left hand and carry the body over the horse to the
left with the right flank towards the horse, and alight on the
ground on the off side of the horse.

Let go with the left hand as soon as you can after you
spring, keep the right arm straight, get the weight well over
it, and keep the weight supported on the right arm as long
as you can. Keep the body and legs in a straight line, and
carry the feet as high as you can consistently with there being
no bend at the waist while passing over the horse; the body
and legs should, in their highest position, be quite horizontal.
Alight clear of the horse, neither hand touching it, exactly
opposite the centre of the saddle. You will find it necessary
at first to hollow the back sharply as you pass over the horse,
but this movement should be disguised as far as possible,
and, if the vault is perfectly done, should be hardly perceptible. During the whole vault a plane passing through the
shoulders and feet should be vertical and very nearly parallel
to the horse, though of course this plane will, while the body
is supported on the right arm, turn through a small angle to

the right. Fig. 6 shows this vault; in the figure the hips and feet are, however, a little lower than they should be for absolute perfection. The great difficulties in a flank

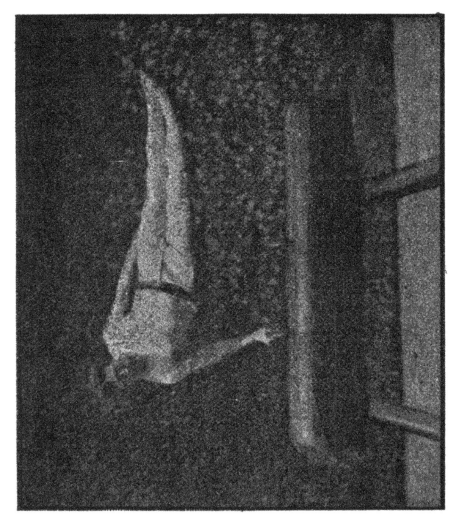

Fig. 6.—FLANK VAULT LEFT.

vault are to get the feet high enough and to alight steadily. Remember, in alighting, *eyes off the ground.*

§ 28. *With a Run, Front Vault Left over Saddle.* Run, spring, and grasp the pommels, as in the last exercise; let go with the left hand and carry the body over the horse to the left with the face towards the horse, alighting on the ground on the off-side of the horse.

Let go with the left hand as soon as you can after you spring, and do a quarter right turn as sharply as possible. Keep the right arm straight and get the weight well over it, and keep the weight supported on the right arm as long as you can; keep the body and legs in a straight line and carry the feet high; the body and legs should, in their highest position, be perfectly horizontal. Alight opposite the croup pommel with the shoulders at right angles to the horse, retaining the grasp of the croup pommel. Fig. 7 shows this vault just before the quarter right turn is completed.

§ 29. *With a Run, Rear Vault Left over Saddle.* Run, grasp the pommels, and spring, as in the last two exercises; let go with the left hand the moment you spring, make a quarter left turn and carry the body over the horse to the left with the back to the horse and the legs horizontal; the moment the legs have passed over the neck pommel, replace the left hand on the pommel and let go with the right hand, hollow the back sharply and alight opposite the croup pommel with the shoulders at right angles to the horse, retaining the grasp with the left hand. During the first part of this vault the back is not hollow, but the legs are nearly at right angles to the body. Fig. 8 shows this vault, which is the easiest vault of the three hitherto described to do well; in the figure the feet are a few inches too high. The only difficulties arc to make the quarter turn soon enough and to avoid ducking the head forward. Lean well back during the first part of the exercise and look well up.

After replacing the left hand on the neck pommel in a rear vault left, you may let go with the left hand again and

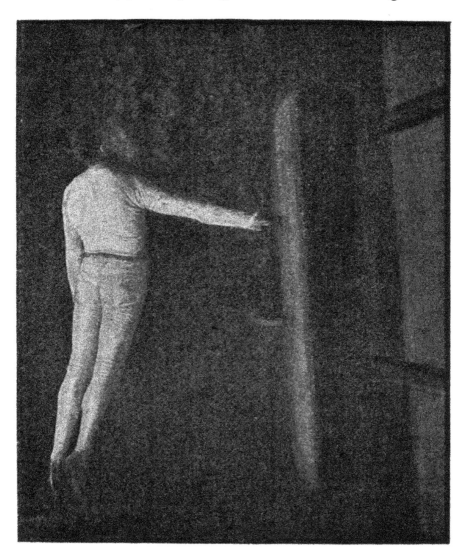

Fig. 7.—FRONT VAULT LEFT.

do a half left turn before you alight, placing the right hand on the neck pommel just before you reach the ground. A half left turn done in this manner after a rear vault left is often called an " inside turn."

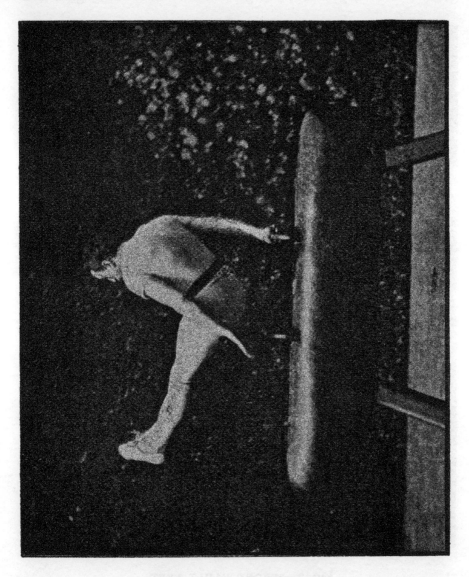

Fig. 8.—REAR VAULT LEFT.

§ 30. *With a Run, Screw Vault Left over Saddle.* Run, grasp the pommels, and spring, as in the last three exercises;

instantly let go with the left hand, throw the right shoulder sharply back, grasp the croup pommel with the left hand, throw the feet as high as possible and carry the body over the horse with, first the left flank, and then the back, to the horse; let go with the right hand and alight opposite the croup pommel with the left hand on the croup pommel; keep the back hollow throughout the exercise. In the course of the vault you make a three-quarter right turn.

This vault is not easy; the great difficulties are to keep the legs together, to keep the back hollow, especially in alighting, and to turn sufficiently early. The vault is not a front vault with a half right turn at the end, but the turning is continuous throughout the vault. When you spring, turn the head and look over the right shoulder.

§ 31. The ordinary vaults, which are eight in number, four right and four left, have now been described. As will be shortly seen, these vaults may be done after various preliminary exercises instead of with a run, accordingly they are often done beginning on the off side and alighting on the near side of the horse. In all the left vaults beginning from the near side and alighting on the off side, the legs pass over the neck and neck pommel; but, if you do a left vault beginning on the off side and alighting on the near side, the legs will pass over the croup and croup pommel. Thus a left vault is always the same movement, *e.g.* in a flank vault left the weight is always supported on the right arm.

I have, in giving the names of the exercises, added the words "over the saddle," because, as will be explained later, vaults may be done over the croup, grasping the croup pommel with the left hand and the croup with the right, or over the neck, grasping the neck pommel with the right hand and the neck with the left. In describing an exercise ending with a vault over the saddle, the words "over saddle" may, however, usually be omitted, because from the position immediately preceding the vault, it will usually be clear that the vault must be done over the saddle.

FEINTS.

§ 32. The movements called feints, which are described in the next few paragraphs, are nothing in themselves, but are of great importance in combination with other exercises. To render my explanation clear, I shall describe them followed by vaults.

§ 33. *From the Front Rest, Right Feint and Flank Vault Left.* From the front rest swing the right leg boldly over the croup and round the right arm, at the same time throwing almost the whole weight on the right arm so that the left arm serves merely to steady the body; let the right leg swing as far as it will go, and then, without pause, swing it back over the croup and, just before it joins the left leg, raise the left leg, so that you are momentarily in the free front rest, and do a flank vault left. The right leg does not touch the horse at all during the exercise; the left leg remains in contact with the horse during the whole feint, but turns as you make the feint, so that when the right leg is at the extremity of its swing the inside of the left thigh is against the horse.

Any of the left vaults may be done after the right feint; the rear vault is the easiest to do well, and the screw vault much the most difficult.

The main difficulties in the right feint are to keep the right leg straight and to avoid touching the horse with it, and, in vaults after the feint, other than the rear vault, to get the body sufficiently high. Fig. 9 shows the right feint just before the right leg is swung to the furthest point.

§ 34. *From the Front Rest, Right Double Feint and Flank Vault Left.* From the front rest swing both legs over the

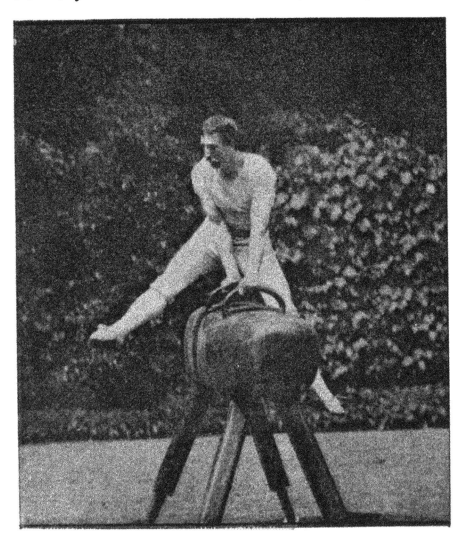

Fig. 9.—RIGHT FEINT.

croup round the right **arm**, keep the legs clear of **the** horse and let them swing **as** far **as** you can, then, without pause, return them and vault left. When the legs are at the extremity of their swing, the left thigh is in contact with the right arm. The double feint is difficult and requires considerable strength; it is easier after a left feint than direct from the front rest. The main difficulties are to keep the legs together in the feint, to avoid touching the horse with them, and to keep them sufficiently high, and, in the subsequent vault, to keep them straight. The right double feint may of course be followed by any left vault. The double feint and screw vault is an exercise which will test the powers of a fine gymnast. Fig. 10 shows the right double feint at the moment when the legs are swung to the furthest point.

§ 35. *From the Front Rest, Right Screw Feint and Flank Vault Left.* From the front rest swing the left leg behind the right and over the croup, at the same time turning the shoulders as far to the left as you can. Swing the left leg as far as it will go, and then, without pause, return it, turning back again to the right; as you approach the front rest again, raise the right leg and do a flank vault left. The left leg does not touch the horse throughout the exercise; the right leg remains in contact with the horse during the whole feint, but turns as you make the feint, so that when the left leg is at the extremity of its swing the outside of the right thigh is against the horse.

The screw feint is not an easy movement, and, at the best, is rather constrained. The right screw feint may of course be followed by any left vault.

§ 36. Each of the expressions, "feint," "double feint," and "screw feint" means a complete movement, beginning from a front rest or free front rest and concluding in a front rest or free front rest. I may point out that the expressions "right feint" and "left feint" are used for other movements

somewhat similar to the feints described in § 33, as will be
explained in § 65. These movements, as will appear,

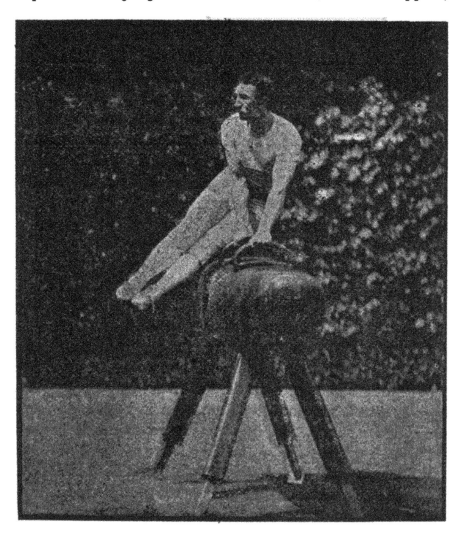

Fig. 10.—RIGHT DOUBLE FEINT.

cannot be done from any position from which the feint
described in § 33 can be done, without some intermediate
movement, so that no confusion is likely to arise in this way.

CIRCLES.

§ 37. *From the Front Rest, Right Circle with Right Leg.*
From the front rest raise the legs to the free front rest, pass
the right leg under the left leg (that is, between the left leg
and the horse) and over the neck pommel, raising the left
hand to let the leg pass ; replace the left hand ; continue
the swing with the right leg and pass it back over the croup
pommel, raising the right hand to let the leg pass ; replace
the right hand and return to the front rest. The left thigh
comes in contact with the horse again as the right leg passes
the neck pommel, and remains in contact with the horse
during the remainder of the exercise.

The main difficulties in this exercise are to keep the right
leg straight and to prevent its touching the horse; you
must keep the weight well over the centre of the horse,
replace each hand in turn as soon as possible after raising
it, shift the weight well to the right while the left hand is
raised and well to the left while the right hand is raised,
and keep the shoulders perfectly square throughout the
movement; do not turn to the left to get the leg over the
neck pommel, nor to the right to get it back again over
the croup pommel. In beginning the exercise, you must
raise the legs sharply from the horse.

§ 38. *From the Front Rest, Right Circle with Left Leg.*
From the front rest carry the left leg over the neck pommel,
raising the left hand, then back over the croup pommel,
raising the right hand, and return to the front rest. The
right thigh remains in contact with the horse until the right
hand is raised; at the moment of raising the right hand the
right leg must be raised from the horse, to make room for
the left leg to pass underneath.

The only particular difficulty about this exercise is to

prevent the right knee bending at the moment of raising the right leg from the horse to let the left leg pass. This is extremely difficult, and, although the bending can be made very slight, it is almost impossible to avoid it altogether.

§ 39. Each of the circles described above may be done with a run, or after a right feint of any kind, and, indeed, after any exercise which brings you to a free front rest. Again, each of these circles may be followed by a left vault of any kind. It is not difficult to do any left vault after a right circle with the right leg, except the screw vault; in doing these exercises the right leg should not touch the horse. It is difficult to do any left vault after a right circle with the left leg, and to do a front or screw vault in this manner is extremely difficult; in these exercises, after the right leg is raised to let the left leg pass, neither leg should touch the horse again.

§ 40. With the movements already described it is easy to construct fairly long exercises of different degrees of difficulty. The following exercise may serve as an example: With a Run, Right Circle with Right Leg, Right Circle with Left Leg, Left Feint, Left Circle with Left Leg, Left Circle with Right Leg, Right Feint, Left Double Feint, and Flank Vault Right.

§ 41. *From the Back Rest, Right Circle with Right Leg.* From the back rest carry the right leg back over the croup pommel, raising the right hand, and then forward over the neck pommel, raising the left hand, and return to the back rest. The left thigh remains in contact with the horse during this circle, until the right leg is passing over the neck pommel, when it is raised to let the right leg pass underneath.

This is not a very easy movement. In beginning, you

must bend at the waist, as explained in § 23, and then, in
order to get a good start, swing both legs a little to the left.
You must keep the swing going freely, and, in bringing the
leg over the neck pommel, throw the weight well to the
right.

§ 42. *From the Back Rest, Right Circle with Left Leg.*
From the back rest pass the left leg under the right, and
over the croup pommel, raising the right hand, then over
the neck pommel, raising the left hand, and return to the
back rest. The right leg must be raised to let the left leg
pass underneath, and does not come in contact with the
horse again till you return to the back rest.

This is not an easy movement. As in the last exercise,
you must bend at the waist before you begin, and, in order
to get a good start, swing the legs slightly to the left.

§ 43. *From the Front Rest, Right Circle with Both Legs.*
From the front rest carry both legs over the neck pommel,
raising the left hand, and back over the croup pommel,
raising the right hand, and return to the front rest. The
legs do not touch the horse in this exercise after you leave
the front rest until you return to it.

This exercise is not easy. In carrying the legs over the
neck pommel, keep the right flank to the horse, with the
right hip close to the right hand, and the weight well
on the right arm, replace the left hand as soon as you
can, and shift the weight on to the left arm as quickly as
possible; let the feet drop well down while you are passing through the free back rest, and, in passing the legs
back over the croup pommel, keep the shoulders quite
square, and do not turn at all to the right. It is easier to
do this circle after a right feint than direct from the front
rest.

§ 44. *From the Back Rest, Right Circle with Both Legs.*

From the back rest carry both legs back over the croup pommel, raising the right hand, and then forward over the neck pommel, raising the left hand. In this exercise the legs do not touch the horse after you leave the back rest until you return to the back rest.

This exercise is very difficult. You must bend at the waist at the beginning, and, in order to get a good start, swing the legs slightly to the left, replace the right hand as soon as you can after the legs have passed the croup pommel, and shift the weight on to the right arm as quickly as you possibly can. You must be quick about the whole exercise, and keep the swing going very freely.

§ 45. All the ordinary circles over the saddle have now been described ; they are twelve in number—four right circles with one leg, four left circles with one leg, two right circles with both legs, and two left circles with both legs. The two right circles with both legs, however, are not completely different movements ; in both you carry the legs forwards over the neck pommel in the same manner, and in both you carry the legs backwards over the croup pommel in the same manner ; the only difference is that in one you begin by carrying the legs forwards, and in the other by carrying the legs backwards. In the same way the two left circles with both legs are not completely different movements. Strictly speaking, therefore, there are only ten completely different circles over the saddle.

§ 46. The general distinction between right and left circles is simply that in all right circles the movement of · the circling leg or legs is with the hands of a watch, and, in all left circles against the hands of a watch, the watch being face upwards. In all my explanations of circles I have supposed that the right hand is on the croup pommel, and the left on the neck pommel ; but if in the course of a

D

combination you have turned round so that you are facing the spring-board, nevertheless right circles are with the hands of a watch, and left circles the other way, so that a right circle always remains the same movement.

§ 47. I have hitherto spoken of complete circles, the circling leg or legs passing first over one pommel, and then over the other. You may, however, do only half of any of the circles hitherto described, carrying the circling leg or legs over one pommel only; these movements are called "half circles." Thus, from the front rest a half right circle over the saddle with one leg will bring you to the side riding rest; from that position another half right circle over the saddle with the same leg will bring you back to the front rest; again, from the back rest a half right circle over the saddle with one leg will bring you to the side riding rest, and from that position another half right circle over the saddle with the same leg will bring you to the back rest again.

Half circles may be done not only over the saddle, but also over the neck or croup, and half circles over the saddle may be done which differ slightly from those described in this paragraph; but unless the contrary appears, the expression "half circle" means a half circle over the saddle, done in the manner explained above.

§ 48. All the circles can be done continuously round and round. If from the back rest you do continuous left circles with the right leg, or continuous right circles with the left leg, neither leg touches the horse at all. In all the other continuous circles with one leg, the leg which is not circling rests lightly against the horse during the greater part of the movement, only being raised for a moment to let the circling leg pass; the circling leg, on the other hand, never touches the horse at all.

In the continuous circle with both legs, the legs do not touch the horse at all. You will find it easiest to begin the continuous right circle with both legs, with a right feint. As the legs pass over the neck pommel, keep the right hip close to the right arm, let the hips turn just a little to the left so that the right leg is a little in front of the left as the legs pass over, check your swing as much as you can after the legs have passed the neck pommel, replace the left hand as soon as you can, and shift the weight as quickly as possible on to the left arm, so that the weight is well on the left arm before you quite reach the free back rest; then, the moment you get the weight on to the left arm, swing the legs as fast as you can to the right. As the legs pass back over the croup pommel you must not turn the shoulders at all to the right, but keep them perfectly square. After the legs pass back over the croup pommel you must replace the right hand, and shift the weight on to it as quickly as you can, and keep the swing going very freely till the legs have again passed over the neck pommel.

The continuous circle with both legs is an exercise of great difficulty; but, if you can master it, you will find all other circling exercises fairly easy. The great difficulty is to prevent the legs touching the horse when you are, or rather ought to be, in the free front rest. The secret of the exercise, and indeed of all circling exercises, lies in shifting the weight properly from the one arm to the other.

§ 49. All the circles which I have described as beginning from the front rest may be begun with a run or with a feint, and the various circles can be made to follow each other either directly or with the interposition of a half circle with both legs. The direction of the circles can be reversed by interposing a feint or by reversing the swing while in the free back rest.

§ 50. All the circles which finish in the front rest may be followed by a vault without pause. Right circles with one leg, followed by left vaults, have been already dealt with in § 39. A right circle with both legs may be followed by any left vault; in these exercises the legs never touch the horse at all; they are all difficult movements, and with a front or screw vault, extremely difficult.

§ 51. The following exercise may serve to show the manner in which circles and feints may be combined, and an exercise finished by a vault. The words in parentheses are added to make the exercise doubly clear; they are not necessary in giving a description of the exercise to a gymnast familiar with the nomenclature employed: With a Run, Half Right Circle with Both Legs (this brings you to the free back rest, let the legs swing a little to the right without pausing, and continue), Left Circle with Right Leg (bringing you again to the free back rest), Half Left Circle with Both Legs, Double Feint Right, Right Circle with Right Leg (the left leg comes in contact with the horse as the left hand is raised; if the exercise is properly done this is the first time either leg touches the horse); Right Circle with Both Legs and Front Vault Left (the left leg, which we left in contact with the horse, is raised just before the right circle with the right leg is complete, and after that the horse is not touched again with either leg).

§ 52. All the vaults and circles can be done starting from various seats on the croup or neck; thus—

(i.) From the Riding Seat on Croup facing Neck, Left Vault or Right Circle over Saddle. Come to the riding seat on the croup facing the neck, grasp the pommels in the usual way, raise the weight on the right arm, and you will be nearly in the same position as if you were doing a right feint, then do any left vault or right circle in the same way as after a right feint. Do not pause after raising the weight, but do the exercise in one movement, so that you appear to start directly from the seat.

(ii.) From the Cross Seat on the Off Side of Croup, Left Vault or Right Circle over Saddle. Come to the cross seat mentioned, grasp the pommels as in the last exercise, raise the weight on the right arm, and you will be nearly in the same position as if you were doing a right double feint; then, without pause, do a left vault or right circle. Do not pause after raising the weight, but do the whole exercise in one movement.

(iii.) From the Side Riding Seat on Croup Facing the Spring-board with Right Leg Forward, Left Vault or Right Circle over Saddle. Come to the seat mentioned, grasp the pommels as in the last exercise, raise the weight on the right arm, and you will be nearly in the same position as if you were doing a right screw feint; then do a left vault or circle as if from a screw feint. Do not pause in the feint, but do the whole exercise in one movement. You may start the swing in this exercise before you grasp the neck pommel; delaying the grasp with the left hand in this way makes the exercise rather easier.

§ 53. After a right circle from the front rest with either leg, you may, instead of returning to the rest when the circling leg has passed the croup pommel, alight on the spring-board.

(i.) Replacing the right hand and alighting facing the horse.

(ii.) Without replacing the right hand, making a quarter right turn. In doing this movement after the circle with the left leg, you must hollow the back sharply as soon as the left leg is over the croup pommel.

(iii.) Without replacing the right hand on the croup

pommel, making a quarter left turn, letting go with the left hand, and grasping the neck pommel with the right hand.

§ 54. After a right circle with either leg from the back rest, you may, instead of coming to the back rest, alight on the ground—

(i.) Without a turn. In this case do not replace the left hand, and you will alight nearly as if you had done a flank vault.

(ii.) With a quarter right turn. Do not replace the left hand, and you will alight nearly as if you had done a front vault.

(iii.) With a quarter left turn. Replace the left hand, at the same moment let go with the right hand and hollow the back sharply; you will then alight almost as if you had done a rear vault.

(iv.) With a three-quarter left turn. Replace the left hand, then let go with both hands and make the turn, placing the right hand on the neck pommel just before you reach the ground. This turn, like a similar turn after a rear vault, is often called an "inside turn."

§ 55. You may alight after a circle with both legs; if you alight on the off side of the horse, it will come to the same thing as if you had done a vault. Observe, however, that, if you do a half *right* circle from the front rest to the ground, it comes to the same thing as a *left* vault.

You may also alight on the spring-board after a right circle with both legs—

(i.) Replacing the right hand and alighting facing the horse.

(ii.) Without replacing the right hand, and making a quarter right turn, at the same time hollowing the back sharply. This is an important movement and constitutes a sort of rear vault backwards, and is often called by that name. The shoulders should turn as soon as the legs are clear of the neck pommel, and the right hand should let go the croup pommel rather sooner than in an ordinary right circle. The back must be sharply hollowed the moment the legs are fairly over the croup pommel. This movement is easier than an ordinary circle with both legs, and in some positions is very much easier.

(iii.) Without replacing the right hand, and making a quarter left turn, at the same time hollowing the back, placing the right hand on the neck pommel, and letting go with the left hand; you will thus do a sort of front vault backwards.

SHEARS.

§ 56. *From the Free Side Riding Rest, Front Shears Right to Riding Seat on Croup.* From the free side riding rest with the left leg forward, swing both legs as hard as you can to the right, let go with the right hand, turn the shoulders sharply through a quarter left turn, carry the right leg over the horse from the near to the off side, and the left leg over the horse from the off to the near side, the right leg passing over the left, and come to the riding seat on the croup.

You will find it advisable in this exercise to begin by swinging both legs to the left as far as you can, in order to get sufficient swing; while thus swinging the legs to the left, keep the line joining the two feet at right angles to the horse.

The main difficulties in this exercise are to swing the legs high enough to the right, and to turn sharply enough so that you come quite squarely to the riding seat. Both thighs should come in contact with the horse simultaneously.

§ 57. *From the Free Side Riding Rest, Front Shears Right*

to Riding Seat in Saddle. Do the same movement as in the last exercise exactly, except that you alight in the saddle instead of on the croup. In order to do this, you have merely to keep the weight more to the left than in the last exercise.

§ 58. *From the Free Side Riding Rest, Front Shears Right.* Do the same movement as in the last exercise, but without turning the shoulders at all, and replace the right hand on the croup pommel, so that you come to a free side riding rest in the saddle with the right leg forward. This exercise might be more fully described as " from the free side riding rest, front shears right to the free side riding rest ; " but, when the expression " front shears " is used alone, it is understood that the exercise finishes in the free side riding rest.

§ 59. You may do front shears right, and, without pausing, continue the swing and do front shears left, and so on, right and left alternately. Neither leg should touch the horse throughout this exercise. You must keep the legs as far apart as possible while passing through the free side riding rest, swing as high to each side as you possibly can, replace each hand in turn, after raising it, as soon as possible, and then shift the weight on to it as quickly as you can. This is an exercise of great difficulty, but will repay constant practice.

§ 60. *From the Free Side Riding Rest, Back Shears Right to Riding Seat on Croup.* From the free side riding rest with the right leg forward swing both legs to the right as hard as you can, let go with the right hand, pass the right leg over the horse from the off to the near side and the left leg over the horse from the near to the off side, the right leg passing over the left ; turn the shoulders sharply, though a quarter right turn, and come to the riding seat on the croup facing outwards. In this exercise you will find it advisable to begin by swinging both legs as far as you can to the left in order to get a good swing; while thus swinging the legs to the left, keep the line joining the feet at right angles to the horse.

§ 61. *From the Free Side Riding Rest, Back Shears Right to Riding Seat in Saddle.* Do the same movement as in the last exercise, coming to the riding seat in the saddle; this is rather easier than the last exercise.

§ 62. *From the Free Side Riding Rest, Back Shears Right.* Do the same movement as in the last exercise, but without turning the shoulders at all, and replace the right hand on the croup pommel, so that you come to the free side riding rest in the saddle with the left leg forward. This exercise might be more fully described as " from the free side riding rest, back shears right to the free side riding rest;" but, when the expression " back shears " is used alone, it is understood that you are to finish in the free side riding rest.

§ 63. You may do back shears right and, without pausing, continue the swing and do back shears left, and so on, right and left alternately. This is an exercise of extreme difficulty, and I have never seen it done quite satisfactorily. It is comparatively easy to do back shears twice in succession, but it is extremely difficult to prevent the swing dying away after that.

§ 64. The distinction between front shears and back shears is that, in front shears, the leg which passes over the other moves forward, whereas, in back shears, the leg which passes over the other moves backwards. Both front and back shears may be combined with the various circles in various ways. The secret of these combinations lies in getting the leg which is not circling immediately before the shears, swung to the left, if you are going to do shears right, and to the right if you are going to do shears left, and in keeping the shoulders perfectly square. For example—

(i.) From the Front Rest, Right Circle with Left Leg, Half Right Circle with Left Leg, and Front Shears Right. In this exercise, as the left leg is moving over the neck pommel for the second time, swing the right leg as far as you can to the left, so that while the left leg swings back to the right the right leg swings with it.

(ii.) From the Front Rest, Half Right Circle with Both Legs, Half Right Circle with Right Leg, and Back Shears Left. In this exercise, as the right leg passes over the croup pommel, swing the left leg well to the right, so that while the right leg swings to the left the left leg swings with it.

The following exercise will serve to show how circles and shears may be combined: With a Run, Half Right Circle with Left Leg, Front Shears Right, Half Right Circle with Left Leg (coming to the free back rest), Half Right Circle with Right Leg, Back Shears Left, Half Right Circle with Right Leg, Half Right Circle with Both Legs, Half Left Circle with Right Leg (reversing the swing in the free back rest), Front Shears Right, Half Right Circle with Left Leg, and Rear Vault Backwards alighting on the Spring-board.

EXERCISES WITH REST ASTRIDE ONE ARM.

§ 65. The exercises described in the next two paragraphs introduce a new kind of feint and a new position. If you are in a side riding rest in the saddle with the left leg forward and are directed to make a "right feint," you must carry the right leg over the croup till you reach a position in which the legs are astride the right arm. This position is called the "rest astride the right arm," or the "free rest astride the right arm," according as. the legs do or do not touch the horse. From a side riding rest with the right leg forward, a left feint will of course bring you to a rest or free rest astride the left arm. In a rest or free rest astride one arm, the feet should nearly touch each other. The free rest astride the right arm is shown in Fig. 11.

§ 66. From the rest or free rest astride the right arm you may carry the right leg back over the croup, coming to a side riding rest, from which you may continue as you please. The following exercises introduce this movement.

(i.) From the Front Rest, Half Right Circle with Left Leg, Feint Right, Half Right Circle with Right Leg over Croup, and Half Right Circle with Right Leg over Saddle to Back Rest. In this exercise, after the half right circle with the left leg, carry the right leg over the croup, coming to the free rest astride the right arm, then return the right leg over the croup and do a half right circle with the right leg, coming to the back rest ; after you reach the free rest astride the right arm, you must, without pause, let the legs move a little to left and then back again, and, without checking the swing, carry the right leg back over the croup.

(ii.) From the Back Rest, Half Left Circle with Right Leg, Right Feint, Half Right Circle with Right Leg over Croup, and Back Shears Left.

§ 67. From the rest or free rest astride the right arm, you may do a half left circle with the left leg, which will bring you to a position similar to that which you reach when the right leg has been carried over the croup in a right feint from the front rest ; you may then return the right leg over the croup and proceed as if you had done an ordinary right feint, or you may continue the swing with the left leg and carry it over the croup. The following exercises introduce this movement.

(i.) From the Front Rest, Half Right Circle with Left Leg, Right Feint, Half Left Circle with Left Leg, Half

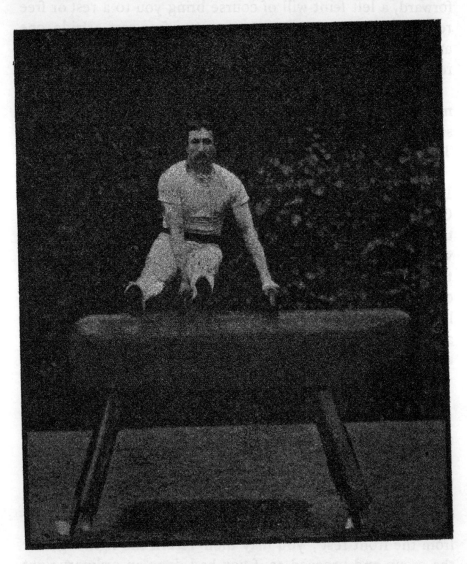

Fig. II.—FREE REST ASTRIDE THE RIGHT ARM.

Left Circle with Left Leg over Croup to join Right Leg, Return Both Legs over Croup, and continue as you please.

In this exercise, when you reach the free rest astride the right arm, do a half left circle with the left leg, continue the swing, and carry the left leg over the croup to join the right, you are then in exactly the position you reach in a right double feint; return the legs over the croup, as in a double feint, and continue as you please. You should not pause at all in the free rest astride the right arm in this exercise, but, the moment the position is reached, swing the left leg to the left.

(ii.) From the Free Rest Astride Right Arm, Half Left Circle with Left Leg and Back Shears Right. In this exercise, after the half left circle with the left leg, you proceed almost as if you intended to do a half left circle with the left leg over the croup to join the right leg, as in the last exercise; but, just before the half circle over the croup is complete, carry the right leg back over the croup and over the left leg, let go with the right hand, and come to the side riding rest in the saddle with the left leg forward.

EXERCISES OVER THE NECK AND CROUP.

. § 68. Exercises exactly similar to those already described may be done over the croup instead of over the saddle, the one hand being placed on the croup pommel and the other on the croup. The hand which is placed on the croup should be at a distance from the croup pommel about equal to the distance between the pommels, with the fingers pointing straight across the horse in the direction in which you are facing; the tendency at first is to get this hand too far from the croup pommel and turned outwards so that the fingers point nearly towards the croup; this tendency you must be careful to check. The hand on the croup pommel should grasp the pommel in the centre.

Exercises may, of course, also be done over the neck; but

these it is unnecessary to discuss, as they correspond exactly with the exercises over the croup.

Exercises over the croup may, of course, be begun from various rests on the croup, and some of them also with a run ; it remains to point out how these exercises may be combined with the exercises over the saddle already explained. I must, however, in the next two paragraphs, premise a few words about the grasp, and about the meaning of certain expressions. Then, in §§ 71–100, I shall describe various ways of combining exercises over the croup with exercises over the saddle.

§ 69. *The Grasp.* In the exercises hitherto explained, the grasp has presented no difficulty, the right hand has, at the beginning of the exercises, always been on the croup pommel, with the back of the hand towards the croup, the left hand on the neck pommel, with the back of the hand towards the neck. When the pommels are grasped in this way, each hand is said to have the " ordinary grasp," or, more accurately, the ordinary grasp for exercises over the saddle.

If you intend to do exercises over the croup with one hand on the croup pommel, and the other hand on the croup, you will naturally grasp the croup pommel with the back of the hand towards the neck, and, in that position, the hand on the croup pommel is said to have the ordinary grasp for exercises over the croup.

You may, however, do exercises over the saddle with the right hand turned through a half left turn from the ordinary grasp, in which case the right hand is said to have a " reverse grasp" for exercises over the saddle. Similarly you may do exercises over the saddle with the left hand turned through a half right turn from the ordinary grasp, in which case the left hand is said to have a reverse grasp for exercises over the saddle.

Again, you may do exercises over the croup facing the off side of the horse, with the left hand grasping the croup pommel and turned through a half right turn from the ordinary grasp, in which case the left hand is said to have the reverse grasp for exercises over the croup; or, facing the near side of the horse, with the right hand on the croup pommel and turned through a half left turn from the ordinary grasp, in which case the right hand is said to have the reverse grasp for exercises over the croup.

If, from the back rest on the saddle with ordinary grasp, you let go with the left hand, do a half right turn, and place the left hand on the croup, you will come to the front rest on the croup with the right hand in reverse grasp for exercises over the croup ; again, if, from the front rest on the saddle with the right hand in reverse grasp, you let go with the left hand, do a half left turn, and place the left hand on the croup, you will come to the back rest on the croup with the right hand in ordinary grasp for exercises over the croup.

§ 70. *Meaning of Expressions " Circle" and " Half Circle."* In doing any of the half circles over the saddle, discussed in § 47, you begin with one hand on each pommel and raise one hand in the course of the half circle ; in similar movements over the croup, you begin with one hand on the croup pommel and the other on the croup, and raise one hand in the course of the half circle. You may, however, do half circles beginning with the hands in some other position ; you then do the same movement with the circling leg or legs as in an ordinary half circle, but, unless the contrary appears, you retain the grasp you had at the beginning of the movement. The expression "half circle" has already been used with the last explained meaning in the description of some of the exercises given in §§ 66, 67. As an additional example of the use of the expression with this meaning, I may point out that a right feint from the front rest might be described as "from the front rest, half left circle over croup with right leg and half right circle over croup with right leg."

Again, in doing any of the circles over the saddle, described in §§ 37-46, you begin with one hand on each pommel and raise each hand in turn in the course of the circle; and, in similar movements over the croup, you begin with one hand on the croup pommel and one hand on the croup, and raise each hand in turn. You may, however, do circles beginning with the hands in some other position; you then do the first half circle in the manner described above, retaining the original grasp, and then take such a grasp as will enable you to complete the circles in the ordinary manner. These explanations seem intricate; practically, however, you will find no difficulty in following the description of any particular exercise, in which the expressions "circle" and "half circle" occur, with the meanings explained above.

EXERCISES OVER CROUP FROM RIDING SEAT ON SADDLE.

§ 71. From the riding seat on the saddle facing the croup, you may do circles or vaults over the croup. For example—

(i.) From the Riding Seat on Saddle facing Croup, Left Vault over Croup. In the riding seat mentioned, grasp the croup pommel with the right hand, with the back of the hand to the body, so that you have the ordinary grasp for exercises over the croup, place the left hand on the croup, raise the weight on the right arm, swing the right leg backwards over the saddle, and vault over the croup. This exercise is precisely similar to those described in § 52, except that you start on the saddle and vault over the croup, instead of starting on the croup and vaulting over the saddle.

(ii.) From the Riding Seat on Saddle facing Croup, Right Circle with Both Legs over Croup, and Quarter Right Turn to Ground. This is little more than a continuation of the last exercise ; you finish with a rear vault backwards, as explained in § 55. If you do a right circle with both legs over the croup facing the near side of the horse, or a left circle with both legs over the croup facing the off side of the horse, it is much easier to finish with the rear vault backwards than to grasp the pommel again and come to the front rest, because the sharp hollowing of the back will help to raise the legs over the pommel.

(iii.) From the Riding Seat on Saddle facing Croup, Right Circle with Right Leg over Croup, Half Right Circle with Both Legs over Croup, Half Left Circle with Right Leg over Croup to Riding Seat on Croup. Continue with movements over the saddle, as in the exercises described in § 52.

CHANGES BETWEEN SADDLE AND CROUP, WITH REST ASTRIDE ONE ARM.

§ 72. From the rest astride the right arm, you may do a half right circle over the croup with the right leg, at the same time letting go with the left hand, turning to the right, and placing the left hand on the croup. You will then be in the same position as if you were doing a right feint preparatory to exercises over the croup, but the right hand will be reversed for these exercises ; if you only propose to vault over the croup, you may keep the right hand in this position, and make your vault, and it is possible to make more complicated movements without changing the grasp until the right hand has to be raised. Having the right hand in this

E

position, however, will add immensely to the difficulty; it is better, therefore, as a rule, to change the grasp of the right hand to the ordinary grasp for exercises over the croup, the moment the left hand is placed on the croup; you will then be exactly in the same position as if you were doing a right feint, and may make such circles as you like over the croup. You will find some difficulty in keeping the swing going during this change of grasp, but it can be done. The following exercise introduces this movement: From the Front Rest, Half Right Circle with Left Leg, Right Feint, Half Right Circle with Right Leg over Croup, Turning to the Right and Placing Left Hand on Croup, Change Right Hand to Ordinary Grasp, Half Right Circle with Right Leg over Saddle, Right Circle with Left Leg over Croup, and Alight with Quarter Left Turn.

§ 73. A movement exactly similar to that described in the last paragraph may be made, which will enable you to proceed with exercises over the saddle after exercises over the croup. The following exercise introduces this movement: From the Back Rest on Near Side of Croup, Half Left Circle with Right Leg over Croup, Feint Right (bringing you to the rest astride the right arm with the left hand on the croup), Half Right Circle with Right Leg over Saddle, Turning to the Right and Placing Left Hand on Neck Pommel, Change Right Hand to Ordinary Grasp, Half Right Circle with Right Leg over Croup, Right Circle with Both Legs over Saddle and Flank Vault Left to Ground.

§ 74. From the free rest astride the right arm you may let go with the left hand and do a half right turn, keeping the legs astride the right arm, with the feet close together, and carrying them over the croup, and then place the left hand on the croup to the left of the left leg; with this movement you reach a rest astride the right arm with the left hand on the croup and with the right hand in reverse grasp, and you may continue accordingly, either retaining the reverse grasp with the right hand, or changing to ordinary grasp the moment you place the left hand on the croup. The movement just described is called a " half right circle with both legs astride the right arm." The following exercise introduces this movement: From the Front Rest, Half Right Circle with Left Leg, Feint Right, Half Right Circle with Both Legs Astride the Right Arm, Place Left Hand on Croup, Change Right Hand to Ordinary Grasp, Half Right Circle with Right Leg over Saddle, and Half Right Circle with Right Leg over Croup, and alight or continue as you please. This exercise, after the half circle with the legs astride the right arm is completed, is like those described in § 66.

§ 75. A movement exactly similar to that described in the last paragraph may be made, which will enable you to proceed with exercises over the saddle after exercises over the croup. This movement corresponds to that described in the last paragraph, just as the movement described in § 73 corresponds to that described in § 72.

§ 76. From the free rest astride the right arm with the right hand in reverse grasp, you may let go with the left hand and do a half left turn, keeping the legs astride the right arm, with the feet close together, and carrying them over the saddle, and then place the left hand on the croup to the left of the left leg; in this way you reach a rest astride the right arm with the left hand on the croup, and you may continue accordingly. The movement just described is called a "half left circle with both legs astride the right arm." It is the reverse of the movement described in § 74. The following exercise introduces this movement: From the Free Rest Astride Right Arm with Right Hand in Reverse Grasp, Half Left Circle with Both Legs Astride Right Arm, Place Left Hand on Croup, Half Left Circle with Left Leg over Croup, and Half Left Circle with Left Leg over Saddle to join Right Leg, Half Right Circle with Both Legs over Saddle, and Rear Vault Left over Croup to Ground.

§ 77. A movement exactly similar to that described in the last paragraph may be made, which will enable you to proceed with exercises over the saddle after exercises over the croup. The following exercise introduces this movement: From the Free Rest Astride the Right Arm, Facing the Near Side of Horse, with Right Hand on Croup Pommel in Reverse Grasp, and Left Hand on Croup, Half Left Circle with Both Legs Astride Right Arm, Place Left Hand on Neck Pommel, Half Left Circle with Left Leg over Saddle and Back Shears Right to Riding Seat on Saddle. The movements, after the half circle with both legs astride the right arm, in this exercise, and in the exercise given in § 76, are like those described in § 67.

EXERCISES OVER CROUP FROM SEATS ON NECK.

§ 78 From the riding seat on the neck facing the croup, you may place both hands on the croup pommel, and do right vaults over the croup; you must swing the left leg sharply back over the neck, carry both legs past the saddle without touching the horse with them, and then carry the legs over the croup, letting go with the right hand.

For the rear vault, you should grasp the pommel with the backs of both hands up; for the flank or front vault, you must grasp the pommel with the back of the right hand up and the palm of the left up, so that the left hand has the ordinary grasp for exercises over the croup, and the right hand has ordinary grasp for exercises over the saddle.

These movements seem very difficult at first, but are not really so; you must keep the weight well to the left from the beginning of the movement, keep the left arm straight, and pull strongly as you begin the movement, especially with the right arm.

§ 79. From the riding seat on the neck facing the croup, you may place both hands on the croup pommel, and do a half left circle with one leg or both legs over the croup, and continue as you please. You must take the same grasp of the croup pommel as you would for a flank vault over the croup, as explained in the preceding paragraph ; then swing the left leg back over the neck, and carry one leg or both legs over the croup ; place the right hand on the croup, so that you reach a back rest or a side riding rest on the croup, from which positions you may continue with various movements.

§ 80. From the riding seat on the neck facing the croup, you may place both hands on the croup pommel, and do a half left circle with both legs over the croup, as explained in the last paragraph, and, without placing the right hand on the croup, turn to the left, shift the right hand to the neck pommel, and come to the front rest on the off side of the saddle with the left hand in reverse grasp.

§ 81. Right vaults and left half circles over the croup may be done in a manner similar to that explained in the last three paragraphs, from the cross seat on the neck with the legs on either the near side or off side of the horse, also from a side riding seat on the neck facing the near side of the horse with the left leg forward.

DOUBLE REAR VAULTS AND SIMILAR MOVEMENTS

§ 82. After any right circle or half circle over the saddle, which would naturally bring you to a back rest, you may, without replacing the left hand on the neck pommel, continue with a right circle or half circle, with one or both legs, over the croup. These movements are explained in §§ 83–95 with some detail.

§ 83. *From the Side Riding Rest on Saddle with Right Leg Forward, Half Right Circle with Left Leg over Saddle, and, Without Replacing Left Hand, Half Right Circle with Left Leg over Croup, to Riding Seat on Croup.* From the side riding rest mentioned, swing the left leg over the neck pommel; when you raise the left hand, throw the left shoulder rather forward and throw the left hand straight above the head, keep the weight on the right arm and keep the right thigh against the horse, roll round on the right thigh and carry the left leg over the croup, coming to the riding seat on the croup facing the neck. This movement is easy; you must do the exercise rather slowly, keep the weight well balanced on the right arm, and keep the right shoulder down.

§ 84. *From the Side Riding Rest on Saddle with Right Leg Forward, Half Right Circle with Left Leg over Saddle, and, Without Replacing Left Hand, Right Circle with Left Leg over Croup, continuing as you please.* Proceed as in the exercise explained in the last paragraph, except that you do not throw the hand above the head; but, when the left leg has just passed over the croup, place the left hand on the croup, complete the circle with the left leg, and either alight or continue with circles over the croup.

§ 85. *From the Front Rest, Half Right Circle with Both*

Legs over Saddle, and, Without Replacing Left Hand, Right Half Circle, or Circle, with Left Leg over Croup. As you do the half right circle with both legs throw the weight well to the right, and, as the legs pass over the neck pommel, throw the left shoulder well forward, then let the right thigh come in contact with the horse, and roll round on the right thigh, keeping the weight on the right arm, carry the left leg over the croup, and, either come to the riding seat, or place the left hand on the croup and continue circling with the left leg over the croup. The left hand is, of course, not replaced on the neck pommel after the legs have passed. If you intend to come to the riding seat you should throw the left hand straight above the head.

§ 86. *From the Front Rest, Half Right Circle with Both Legs over Saddle, and, Without Replacing Left Hand, Half Right Circle with Right Leg over Croup, to Riding Seat on Croup.* Begin as in the exercise described in the preceding paragraph, but turn the shoulders still earlier to the right, and, without letting the legs touch the horse at all, carry the right leg over the croup, and come to the riding seat on the croup facing outwards. This exercise seems difficult at first, but is not really so; you must not be too slow about it. When you raise the left hand, throw the arm forward, look over the right shoulder, and make up your mind that you will not catch hold of the neck pommel again.

§ 87. You may do exercises similar to that described in the last paragraph, but, instead of coming to the riding seat, continue the circle with the right leg, placing the left hand on the croup as soon as the right leg has passed.

§ 88. *From the Front Rest, Half Right Circle with Both Legs over Saddle, and, Without Replacing Left Hand, Rear Vault Left over Croup.* This exercise is very like that explained in § 86, except that, instead of carrying the right leg over the croup, you carry both legs over and alight; once you have learnt the exercise described in § 86, the present exercise will present little difficulty. The moment you let go with the left hand, get the left shoulder well forward, look over the right shoulder, and lean well to the right. The whole movement is often called the double rear vault, or, for greater accuracy, the double rear vault over the saddle and croup. It is a most important exercise to learn. You may, of course, do a similar exercise concluding with a half right circle with both legs to the back rest, instead of with a rear vault.

§ 89. *From the Front Rest, Half Right Circle with Both Legs over Saddle, and, Without Replacing Left Hand, Right Circle with Both Legs over Croup to Ground with a Quarter Right Turn.* Begin as in the exercise described in the last paragraph, but, as soon as the legs have passed over the croup, place the left hand on the croup, and complete the circle, alighting with a quarter right turn. The last half circle is a rear vault backwards, as explained in § 55. The whole exercise is sometimes called a treble rear vault, and makes a very effective conclusion to many exercises; but it is not at all easy. It makes a peculiarly effective finish after continuous right circles with both legs; but this is, of course, an exercise of very great difficulty.

§ 90. *From the Front Rest, Half Right Circle with Both Legs over Saddle, and Without Replacing Left Hand, Right Circle with Both Legs over Croup, and continue with other Right Circles over the Croup.* These exercises begin like that explained in the last paragraph, but, instead of coming to the ground, you keep the shoulders parallel to the horse, replace the right hand on the croup pommel, and continue. These movements are of extreme difficulty; indeed,

I do not think I have ever seen them satisfactorily accomplished. However, they are clearly possible, and I have seen closely analogous exercises accomplished, beginning with circles over the croup, and continuing over the saddle in the manner explained in § 94.

§ 91. *From the Side Riding Rest on Saddle with Right Leg Forward, Half Right Circle with Left Leg; and, Without Replacing Left Hand, Rear Vault Left, or Half Right Circle with Both Legs, or with Right Leg, over Croup, continuing as you please.* These exercises are begun like those explained in §§ 83, 84, but, instead of rolling round on the right thigh, you must raise the right leg, and continue as in the exercises explained in §§ 86–90.

§ 92. *From the Side Riding Rest on Saddle with Left Leg Forward, Half Right Circle with Right Leg, and, Without Replacing Left Hand, continue as in the exercises explained in § 85.* These exercises require no special explanation, and are not very difficult.

§ 93. *From the Side Riding Rest on Saddle with Left Leg Forward, Half Right Circle with Right Leg, and, Without Replacing Left Hand, continue as in the exercises explained in §§ 86–90* These exercises are very difficult. The secret is to turn the shoulders rather late.

§ 94. Exercises similar to those explained in §§ 83–93 may be done, beginning with circles over the croup, and continuing with exercises over the saddle. You will have no difficulty in perceiving how to manage this. The actual change from the croup to the saddle is a good deal more difficult than the corresponding change from the saddle to the croup. On the other hand, after the change is made, it is easier to continue with circles over the saddle than to continue with circles over the croup after the corresponding change from the saddle to the croup.

§ 95. The exercises described in §§ 82–94 may be easily brought into combination with other exercises. In all these exercises the weight has to be carried by the right arm alone for a considerable space of time; accordingly you must, in doing them, get well balanced over the right arm, and, for this purpose, it is most essential to keep the right hip almost in contact with the right arm throughout the movement. Such of these movements as begin in the side riding rest may also, after a suitable preparatory movement, be done from a free side riding rest. In doing the exercises described in § 91 in this manner from a free side riding rest, it is not necessary to let the right leg come in contact with the horse after the half right circle with the left leg, and before doing the remainder of the movement; but you will find it much easier to accomplish these movements if you do let the leg touch the horse, and then raise it sharply.

It should be pointed out that after any right circle or half circle over the saddle, which would naturally bring you to the back rest, you may, without replacing the left hand on the neck pommel, do a half right turn, and come to a front rest on the croup. These exercises are very easy; but may sometimes be introduced effectively.

CHANGES BETWEEN SADDLE AND CROUP, WITH HALF CIRCLE WITH BOTH LEGS, WITH LEGS STRADDLED.

§ 96. A very pretty change may be effected by means of a half circle with both legs, done with the legs straddled. The following exercise introduces this movement: With a Run, Grasp Pommels with Right Hand in Reverse Grasp, Half Left Circle with Both Legs over Croup with Legs Straddled and Back Hollow, Let go with Left Hand, Place Left Hand on Croup, Half Left Circle with Right

Leg over Saddle, and continue as you please. Run, grasp the neck pommel with the left hand in ordinary grasp, and the croup pommel with the right hand in reverse grasp, spring and instantly straddle the legs wide, carry the legs over the croup, keeping the back hollow, the body horizontal, and the face to the horse, at the same time letting go with the left hand. When the legs are clear of the croup, place the left hand on the croup, continue the swing of the body until the right leg comes over the saddle, then slightly drop the legs and raise the shoulders, and you will be in the same position as if doing a right feint preparatory to exercises over the croup; you may continue accordingly.

You may do a similar exercise from the front rest, beginning with a left feint, and reversing the grasp of the right hand as you feint. From the time you have swung the left leg over the neck in the left feint you should keep the legs straddled throughout the movement. Similar exercises may be done from seats on the neck, grasping the neck pommel with the left hand in ordinary grasp, and the croup pommel with the right hand in reverse grasp for exercises over the saddle. These exercises are difficult; you will find it advisable not to tighten the grasp with the right hand until you are fairly started in the swing, as the arm is at first in a very constrained position. Similar exercises may be done after any movement which brings you to a free front rest with the right hand in reverse grasp; but these exercises are of great difficulty. Corresponding exercises may be done bringing you from the croup to the saddle.

CHANGES BETWEEN SADDLE AND CROUP WITH SCREW CIRCLE OR HALF CIRCLE.

§ 97. From the front rest, with the right hand in reverse grasp, you may turn to the left, pass the left leg outside the right leg, and do a left circle or half circle with it over the croup; these circles are called screw circles, or half screw circles. The movement with which they begin is exactly like the movement with which a screw feint is begun. The following exercise introduces a half screw circle: From the Front Rest with Right Hand in Reverse Grasp, Feint Left, Half Left Screw Circle with Left Leg over Croup, Place Left Hand on Croup, and Back Shears Right to Riding Seat on Croup.

§ 98. Screw circles and half screw circles may be done after any left circle or half circle over the saddle, which would naturally bring you to a front rest with the right hand in reverse grasp, without replacing the left hand on the neck pommel. The following exercise introduces this movement: From the Front Rest, Left Circle with Left Leg, Reversing the Grasp of Right Hand as the Left Leg passes over Croup Pommel, and, Without Replacing Left Hand, Left Screw Circle with Left Leg over Croup to Back Rest on Near Side of Croup. From the front rest do a left circle with the left leg; when you replace the right hand, after raising it to let the leg pass, take the reverse grasp with it, and, when you raise the left hand, turn sharply to the left, and, without replacing the left hand on the neck pommel, continue the swing of the left leg, and carry it over the croup, then place the left hand on the croup, and carry the left leg over the croup pommel, raising the right hand, and come to the back rest on the croup facing the spring-board.

CHANGES BETWEEN SADDLE AND CROUP, PLACING BOTH HANDS ON ONE POMMEL.

§ 99. After any left circle or half circle over the saddle, which would naturally bring you to the front rest, you may, instead of replacing the left hand on the neck pommel, place it on the croup pommel, continue the swing, and do a half left circle with one leg or both legs over the croup with both hands on the croup pommel, and then place the right hand on the croup, coming to a back rest or side riding rest on the croup, from which positions you may continue as you please. The following exercises introduce movements of this kind—

(i.) From the Front Rest, Left Circle with Left Leg, Place Left Hand on Croup Pommel, and Left Circle with Right Leg over Croup to Ground with Quarter Left Turn. In this exercise, after the left hand is raised to let the leg pass, do not replace it on the neck pommel, but shift the weight well to the right, and place the left hand on the croup pommel in front of the right hand with the ordinary grasp for exercises over the croup, then swing the right leg over the croup with both hands grasping the right pommel; when the right leg has passed over the croup let go with the right hand, place it on the croup, and continue the circle with the right leg.

(ii.) From the Front Rest, Left Circle with Both Legs, Place Left Hand on Croup Pommel, and Left Circle with Both Legs over Croup to Ground.

§ 100. You may do exercises corresponding to those described in the last paragraph, and bringing you from the croup to the saddle.

TURNS IN SADDLE.

§ 101. From the front rest you may do a half right circle with the left leg, and then do a half right turn, shifting the left hand to the croup pommel and the right hand to the neck pommel, and you may continue with a left feint or a half right circle with the left leg.

This movement should be done without letting the left leg touch the horse, and without pause. The moment you let go with the left hand to let the left leg pass, turn the shoulders very sharply to the right and place the left hand on the croup pommel, checking the swing of the left leg in the meantime, so that, when both hands are on the croup pommel, the left leg is nearer to the neck pommel than to the croup pommel, then turn further to the right and place the right hand on the neck pommel. You may continue with a left feint, which will bring you to a rest astride the left arm; or with a half right circle with the left leg, coming to the back rest or free back rest; or with a half right circle with the left leg, followed, without replacing the left hand, by movements over the neck. The following exercises introduce this turn—

(i.) With a Run, Half Right Circle with Left Leg, Half Right Turn, placing Left Hand on Croup Pommel and Right Hand on Neck Pommel, Left Feint, Half Right Circle over Saddle with Right Leg, Half Right Circle over Croup with Right Leg to join Left Leg, Half Left Circle over Croup with Both Legs, and Double Rear Vault over Saddle and Croup to Ground.

(ii.) From the Front Rest, Right Feint, Half Right Circle with Left Leg, Half Right Turn, Placing Left Hand on Croup Pommel and Right Hand on Neck Pommel, Half Right Circle with Left Leg, and Half Right Circle with Both Legs to Ground with a Quarter Right Turn.

(iii.) From the Front Rest, Right Feint, Half Right Circle with Left Leg, Half Right Turn, Placing Left Hand on Croup Pommel and Right Hand on Neck Pommel, Half Right Circle with Left Leg, and, Without Replacing Left Hand, Right Circle over Neck with Both Legs to Ground with Quarter Right Turn.

(iv.) From the Front Rest, Right Feint, Right Circle with Both Legs, Half Right Circle with Left Leg, Half Right Turn, placing Left Hand on Croup Pommel and Right Hand on Neck Pommel, Half Right Circle with Left Leg, Right Circle with Both Legs, and continue as you please.

§ 102. From the back rest you may do a half right circle with the right leg, then, the moment the right hand is replaced on the croup pommel, turn sharply to the right, place the left hand on the croup pommel, continue the swing of the right leg, and carry it over the neck pommel with both hands on the croup pommel, then turn further to the right and place the right hand on the neck pommel, and continue with a left feint or vault, or with a right circle. This movement must be done without pause and without letting the right leg touch the horse. The following exercise introduces this movement: From the Front Rest, Half Right Circle with Both Legs, Half Right Circle with Right Leg, Quarter Right Turn, Placing Left Hand on Croup Pommel, Half Right Circle with Right Leg, Quarter Right Turn, Placing Right Hand on Neck Pommel, and Right Circle with Both Legs to Ground.

TURNS WITH REST ASTRIDE ONE ARM.

§ 103. From the rest astride the right arm, you may do a half left circle with the left leg over the saddle, and, instead of replacing the left hand on the neck pommel, turn to the left and place it on the croup pommel with the ordinary grasp for exercises over the saddle, then, retaining the grasp of the croup pommel with both hands, do a half left circle with the left leg over the croup, then let go with the right hand, do a half left circle with one leg or both legs over the saddle, turning further to the left, place the right hand on the neck pommel and alight or continue as you please. A similar exercise may be done from a rest astride one arm with the other hand on the croup. The following exercises introduce these movements—

(i.) From the Front Rest, Half Right Circle with Left Leg, Feint Right, Half Left Circle with Left Leg, Placing Left Hand on Croup Pommel, Half Left Circle with Left Leg over Croup, and Left Circle with Both Legs over Saddle to Ground with Quarter Left Turn.

(ii.) From the Front Rest with Right Hand in Reverse Grasp, Half Right Circle with Left Leg, Feint Right, Half Left Circle with Both Legs astride Right Arm, Half Left Circle with Left Leg over Croup, Placing Left Hand on Croup Pommel, Half Left Circle with Left Leg over Saddle, and Rear Vault Right over Croup to Ground.

GENERAL REMARKS.

§ 104. The exercises on the horse which remain to be described differ for the most part considerably in character from those hitherto described, and it will be convenient before passing on to make some general remarks with regard to the latter. Among all these exercises there are six, towards the acquisition of which you should chiefly direct your efforts, namely: Continuous circles with both legs right and left, continuous front shears, continuous back shears, and the double rear vault right and left. If you could do these six exercises properly you would find very little difficulty in any of the movements I have hitherto described. However, I feel bound to admit that you are very unlikely to succeed altogether in accomplishing these exercises, as they are all, except the double rear vaults, of very great difficulty.

It may be of some use to state to what degree of perfection I have actually seen these exercises carried. The finest gymnast I have ever seen does the double rear vault right and left with the greatest ease; he does continuous right circles with both legs eight or ten times round with certainty, and has done twenty such circles; he can generally do continuous left circles with both legs four or five times round, and has done twelve such circles; he does six or eight consecutive front shears with certainty, and has done many more, but he occasionally touches the horse with one leg in the course of the movement; he can generally do two consecutive back shears, and has done four, but the movement always looks forced

SQUATTING MOVEMENTS.

§ 105. *Squatting Movements with a Run.*

(i.) *With a Run, Squat over Saddle to Ground.* Run, grasp the pommels and spring, bend and raise the knees, and carry the body straight over the saddle, letting go the pommels before the legs pass over the horse; as soon as the legs are clear of the horse straighten the knees and hollow the back sharply, so that you assume a vertical position in the air, and alight. You cannot in this movement spring too high or too far. You may vary this exercise by introducing a turn before you alight.

(ii.) *With a Run, Sheep Jump over Saddle to Ground.* Proceed as in the last exercise, but, instead of raising the knees, bend them and carry the feet to the rear, and pass over the horse in this position. This is a difficult movement, but exceedingly pretty. You may introduce a turn after this movement also.

(iii.) *With a Run, Squat over Saddle to Back Rest or Half Lever.* Proceed as in exercise (i.), but retain the grasp,

F

pass the feet between the hands and come to a back rest or half lever.

(iv.) *With a Run, Squat over Saddle with One Leg.* Run, grasp the pommels and spring, bend and raise one knee, and pass the leg over the saddle, coming to a side riding rest.

(v.) *With a Run, Squat over Saddle with Left Leg, and at the Same Time, Half Left Circle over Croup with Right Leg to Rest astride Right Arm.* This exercise requires no description; you must be particularly careful to keep the right leg straight.

§ 106. *Squatting Movements from Front Rest.* The exercises described in the last paragraph may be done from the front rest; but the sheep jump and squat to the ground from the front rest are difficult and ineffective, as it is impossible to do them with sufficient dash to make them look well.

§ 107. *Squatting Movements from Back Rest.* From the back rest you may squat backwards with both legs to a front rest, or to the free front rest, or with one leg to the side riding rest.

§ 108. *Squatting Movements from Side Riding Rest.* From the side riding rest you may squat forwards with the one leg, or backwards with the other; or, forwards with one leg and backwards with the other simultaneously.

§ 109. Squatting movements may be done over the neck or croup instead of over the saddle, either placing one hand on one pommel and the other on the neck or croup; or, placing both hands on the neck or croup. A squat or sheep jump over the croup to the ground with both hands on the croup may be done, turning slightly to the right as you spring, and passing over the horse obliquely. These are rather effective movements.

STRADDLING MOVEMENTS.

§ 110. *With a Run, Straddle over Saddle to Ground.*
Run, grasp the pommels, and spring, straddling the legs as
wide as you can, let go the pommels and pass over the
horse with the legs perfectly straight and straddled wide.
As soon as the legs are over, hollow the back sharply, close
the legs, and alight. The legs should be closed, and the
body and legs quite vertical, some time before you reach
the ground. This is an effective movement, and should be
done with dash. With the horse breast high you should
alight four or five feet from the horse. Fig. 12 shows this
movement just before the back is hollowed. The exercise
may be varied by the introduction of a turn before
alighting.

§ 111. *With a Run, Straddle over Saddle to Back Rest
or Half Lever.* Proceed as in the exercise described in
the last paragraph, but do not hollow the back, and, as soon
as the legs are over, catch the pommels again and come to
the back rest or half lever.

§ 112. *With a Run, Straddle over Saddle and Half
Right Turn to Front Rest.* Proceed as in the exercises
described in the last paragraph, but, the moment the legs
are over the horse, do a half right turn very sharply, catch
the neck pommel with the right hand and the croup
pommel with the left hand, and come to the front rest.

§ 113. The exercises described in the last three paragraphs may also be done from the front rest, but the
straddle to the ground done in this manner is comparatively
ineffective.

§ 114. *With a Run, Back Straddle over Saddle.* Run,
grasp the pommels and spring, instantly let go with both
hands, do a half turn very sharply, straddle the legs, and

pass over the horse backwards with the legs straddled. You may either come to the ground after this movement or

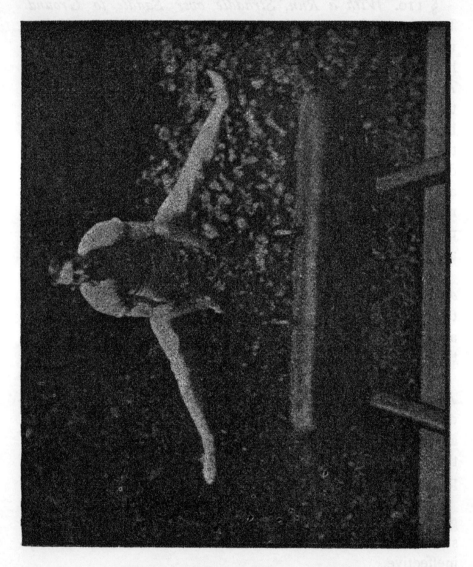

Fig. 12.—STRADDLE OVER SADDLE.

catch the pommels again and come to the front rest on the off side of the horse. The movement is very difficult.

er, and continue as you please.' From the back rest,
at back as explained in § 107, kick the legs sharply

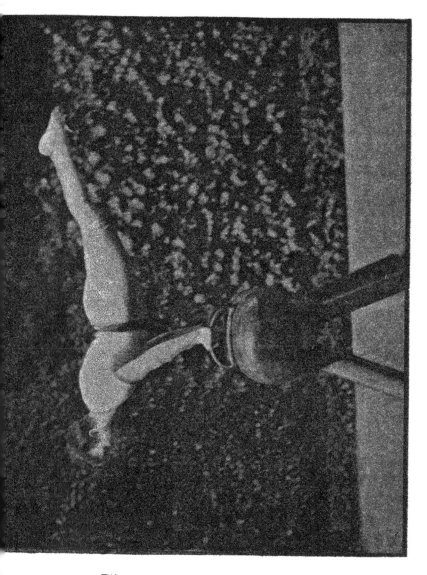

Fig. 13.—FREE FRONT LEVER.

backwards **and** come to the free front lever, then
eed as explained in the **two** preceding paragraphs.

§ 115. *From the Back Rest Straddle E*
Ground. From the back rest, spring from
let go the pommels, straddle the legs wide, p
horse backwards, and alight. This exercise
quite impossible, unless you can straddle
wide ; if you can, it is not difficult.

§ 116. Straddling movements may be done (
or croup instead of over the saddle, either plac
on one pommel and the other on the neck (
placing both hands on the neck or croup. A
the croup, with both hands on the croup, may,
be done obliquely, and a back straddle o
may be done in a somewhat similar manner,
pass over the horse obliquely, and alight aln
the end of the croup. This is an effectiv
and not nearly so difficult as a back strad
saddle.

FRONT LEVER.

§ 117. *Run, Spring to Free Front Lever,*
Back Rest or Half Lever. Run, spring fro
and, after you spring, grasp the pommels, let t
up backwards till you are perfectly horizon
arms straight and the back hollow. Try to r
position for a moment, then bend the knees
legs over the saddle between the hands and
back rest or half lever. Fig. 13 shows t
lever.

§ 118. From the free front lever you ma
the ground, or vault, or do a feint, or dou
squat with one leg. In doing these movemen
show the lever as distinctly as possible before

§ 119. *From the Back Rest, Squat Back t*

The squat backwards to the free front lever, and straddle to ground, is a very effective movement.

THIEF JUMPS.

§ 120. *Run and Thief Jump with One Leg to Side Riding Rest.* Run and spring from one foot, raise the other leg in front of you, keeping it straight, and carry it over the saddle, and, as your body comes over the horse, grasp the pommels. You must spring from a point sufficiently distant from the horse to allow of raising the leg in front of you above the horse without bending it.

§ 121. *Run and Thief Jump with Both Legs to Ground or to Half Lever.* Run and spring from one foot as in the last exercise, carry both feet straight over the saddle in front of you, as if you meant to jump the horse clear, and, as your body comes over the horse, grasp the pommels, and either press at once sharply from the hands and alight or remain in the half lever.

MISCELLANEOUS EXERCISES.

§ 122. You may, with a run, grasp one pommel with both hands, and then, after a circling movement, shift one hand on to the other pommel or on to the neck or croup. These exercises admit of considerable variety. For example—

(i.) You may, with a run, grasp the neck pommel with both hands in ordinary grasp for exercises over the saddle, do a half left circle over saddle with the right leg, or with both legs, or a half left screw circle over the saddle with the left leg, and then place the left hand on the croup pommel and continue.

(ii.) You may, with a run, grasp the neck pommel with both hands in ordinary grasp for exercises over the saddle, do a half left circle over the saddle with both legs, and, without placing the left hand on the croup pommel, do a rear vault right, or a left half circle, or a left circle, over the neck.

(iii.) You may do exercises similar to those last described, taking an ordinary grasp for exercises over the neck with the left hand.

§ 123. You may do exercises similar to those described in the first set of examples given in the last paragraph, taking a grasp of the neck pommel with the right hand only, and not placing the left hand on the horse till the half circle is done.

§ 124. *Wolf Vaults.* You may do flank front or rear vaults over the saddle with the knee of one leg bent, so that one foot passes over the saddle. These movements, which are called "wolf vaults," are at the best rather inelegant; you must keep the leg which is not bent absolutely straight, and bend the other leg a good deal. Corresponding movements may of course be done over the neck or croup.

§ 125. *Fencing Vaults,* etc. You may run and spring from one foot, at the same time grasping one pommel with one hand, and do a flank front or rear vault over the saddle, or over the neck or croup. These vaults are called "fencing vaults." You may also do circling movements, beginning in a similar manner. Right fencing vaults, and left circles beginning in a similar manner, are easier if you spring from the right foot, but they may also be done springing from the left foot.

§ 126. You may, with a run, do a half right circle with both legs over the saddle with a half right turn, letting go with both hands as you pass over the horse, and coming to the front rest, or free front rest, on the off side of the horse. In this exercise, you must let go with both hands simultaneously the moment you spring, pass over the horse with the back hollow and the face towards the horse, and then catch the pommels again with the right hand on the neck pommel and the left hand on the croup pommel. This exercise may be followed by a left vault, or half right circle with both legs, without letting the legs touch the horse.

§ 127. If you grasp the croup pommel with both hands, and rest the toes on the neck, keeping the back hollow, you may spring from the toes and do exercises over the croup in the same manner as from a seat on the neck as described in §§ 78-81.

§ 128. *Handstands.* Handstands on the horse are so similar to the handstands on the horizontal bar and parallel bars described in Chaps. III. and IV., that they need not be discussed at length here. You may reach a handstand on the horse over the saddle with one hand on each pommel, or over the neck or croup with one hand on one pommel and the other on the neck or croup. From the handstand you may do an overthrow, high front vault, squat, or straddle, to ground ; these movements are similar to those on the horizontal bar, described in §§ 249-253. You may lift to the handstand slowly from the front rest, or after squatting backwards slowly from the back rest, or from an elbow lever, and you may sink slowly from the handstand to various positions ; these movements are similar to those on the parallel bars described in §§ 387, 389, 390, 392, 398, 414. You may also run and spring to the handstand ; this movement is similar to the method of reaching the free front lever, described in § 117, but you must, of course, let the legs swing higher; you should endeavour to keep the back hollow throughout this movement.

§ 129. *Elbow Levers.* Elbow levers similar to the elbow

levers on the parallel bars described in §§ 410–412, may be done on the horse. From an elbow lever you may do various exercises similar to those on the parallel bars, described in §§ 410–420. Again, from a right elbow lever you may do left vaults or right circles over the saddle in the same way as from a right feint.

§ 130. *The Needle.* From the front rest, carry the right leg over the croup, turning at the same time to the left; then bend the right knee and pass the right foot over the saddle between the hands from the off side to the near side; then let go with the hands, turn sharply to the left, carry the left leg over the croup and straighten the right knee, coming to the riding seat in the saddle facing the croup.

§ 131. *The Roll Over Backwards to Ground.* From the back rest, let the shoulders drop backwards and let the feet pass over the head; let go with the hands and alight. This movement is similar to the roll over on the parallel bars, described in § 530. The movement should be done as quickly as possible, and you should assume an erect position the instant you alight.

§ 132. Many of the movements described in Part II. of the present chapter may be introduced into exercises on the horse placed sideways; for example—front and back shears from the riding seat, as explained in §§ 137, 138, 183, also all the dismounts explained in §§ 159, 160.

§ 133. *Examples of Combined Exercises.* In the present paragraph I shall give a few combined exercises, placing in parentheses references to the paragraphs in which the particular movements introduced are described, whenever the movement appears at all difficult to follow.

(i.) With a Run, Squat over Saddle with Left Leg, Half Left Circle with Right Leg, Half Left Circle with Left Leg, Half Right Circle with Right Leg, Half Right Circle with

Left Leg, Half Left Circle with Right Leg to Ground with Quarter Right Turn (§ 54). This is thoroughly elementary, but not so easy as it looks to do to perfection.

(ii.) Run, Thief Jump from Left Foot to Side Riding Rest with Right Leg Forward (§ 120), Half Right Circle with Left Leg over Saddle, and, without replacing Left Hand, Half Right Circle with Left Leg over Croup to Riding Seat on Croup (§ 83), Grasp Pommels again with Right Hand on Croup Pommel, Right Circle with Right Leg over Saddle (§ 52), Left Feint, and Rear Vault Right to Ground. This is a fairly easy exercise.

(iii.) With a Run, Right Circle with Right Leg, Left Double Feint, Left Circle with Left Leg, Right Feint, Right Circle with Both Legs, Half Right Circle with Left Leg, Front Shears Right, Front Shears Left to Riding Seat on Neck, Place Both Hands on Croup Pommel, and Rear Vault Right over Croup to Ground. This is an exercise of considerable difficulty.

(iv.) With a Run, Straddle over Saddle to Half Lever, Drop Legs to Back Rest, Squat Back to Free Front Lever, Squat Forward with Left Leg, and, at same time, Half Left Circle with Right Leg over Croup to Rest Astride Right Arm (§ 105, v.), Half Left Circle over Saddle with Left Leg, Back Shears Right (§ 67), Half Left Circle with Left Leg, Right Double Feint, and Screw Vault Left to Ground. This exercise was set at one of the German Gymnastic Society's competitions, and is very difficult to do well.

(v.) With a Run, Right Circle with Right Leg, and without replacing Right Hand on Croup Pommel, Shift Right Hand to Neck Pommel, Right Circle with Both Legs over Neck (§ 99), Half Right Circle with Left Leg over Neck, Right Feint, Half Right Circle with Both Legs astride

Right Arm, Place Left Hand on Croup Pommel, Change
Right Hand to Ordinary Grasp, Half Right Circle with
Right Leg over Neck, and Half Right Circle with Right
Leg over Saddle (§ 66), Right Circle with Both Legs,
and, without replacing Left Hand, Half Right Circle over
Neck with Right Leg to Riding Seat on Neck, Place
Hands on Neck and Dismount with Back Shears (§ 159).
This is an exercise of extreme difficulty.

(vi.) With a Run, Take Reverse Grasp with Right Hand
and Ordinary Grasp with Left Hand, Half Left Circle with
Both Legs over Croup with Legs Straddled and Back
Hollow, Shift Left Hand to Croup, Right Feint (§ 96),
Right Circle over Croup with Both Legs, Half Right Circle
over Croup with Both Legs, and, without replacing Left
Hand, Right Circle with Both Legs over Saddle, Half Right
Circle with Both Legs over Saddle, and, without replacing
Left Hand, Right Circle over Croup with Both Legs to
Ground with Quarter Right Turn.   This exercise I con-
sider the most difficult I have ever seen accomplished.

PART II.—*EXERCISES ON HORSE WITHOUT POM-
MELS, AND ON HORSE PLACED LENGTH-
WAYS.*

§ 134. Preliminary—§ 135. Exercises from Front Rest—
§§ 136–138. Exercises from Riding Seat—§§ 139–
143. Half Circles over Croup with One Leg—§§ 144–
147. Vaults—§ 148. Circles to Front Rest—§§
149–158. Mounts—§§ 159, 160. Dismounts—§§ 161–
168. Long Jumps—§§ 169, 170. Jumps over Croup,
returning to Spring-board—§§ 171–173. Exercises

with Handstand—§§ 174–183. Exercises on Horse placed lengthways with Pommels.

PRELIMINARY.

§ 134. The more important exercises on the horse without pommels are done with the horse placed lengthways, that is, with the spring-board at the end of the horse close to the croup, and throughout the present part of the chapter the horse is supposed to be so placed, unless the contrary appears ; some of the exercises described, however, may also be done with the horse placed sideways.

The word " run " in the description of exercises on the horse placed lengthways, means, run and spring from the spring-board from both feet.

In the front rest on the horse without pommels, you must place the hands well on the further side of the horse from the legs with the fingers over the side of the horse and pointing downwards.

EXERCISES FROM THE FRONT REST.

§ 135. From the front rest you may do flank front or rear vaults, or squatting or straddling movements, half circles with one leg or both legs, and other exercises similar to those described in the first part of the present chapter. These exercises require no particular explanation, they are as like the corresponding exercises on the horse with pommels as may be ; they may, of course, many of them, also be done with a run, with the horse placed sideways.

EXERCISES FROM THE RIDING SEAT.

§ 136. From the riding seat, you may do exercises similar to those described in § 52. If, from a riding seat facing the neck, you intend to do left vaults or right half circles in this manner you must place the hands on the off side of the horse in front of the right leg with the fingers over the side of the horse, at the same time turning the shoulders slightly to the right.

§ 137. *From the Riding Seat, Back Shears with Half Left Turn.* From the riding seat, place the hands in front of you with the fingers pointing forward, and the hands opposite each other, swing the legs up behind you, slightly bending the arms, till the body is clear of the horse and almost horizontal; then do a half left turn sharply, raising the left hand, straddle the legs, raise the right hand, and come to the riding seat. The legs should come in contact with the horse simultaneously, after the right hand is raised. This exercise is not very easy to do well.

§ 138. *From the Riding Seat, Front Shears with Half Left Turn.* From the riding seat, place the hands behind you, one on each side of the horse, with the fingers pointing outwards and downwards, swing the legs up in front as high as you can; as soon as the legs are clear of the horse, do a half left turn sharply, letting go with the right hand, and hollow the back; then straddle the legs, let go with the left hand and come to the riding seat.

HALF CIRCLES TO GROUND WITH ONE LEG.

§ 139. *Run, Hands on Croup, Straddle, and Half Right Circle with Left Leg to Ground.* Run, place the hands on the croup and spring, straddle the legs and carry the left leg over the horse from the near side to the off, raising the hands to let it pass, replace the left hand on the croup and alight with the shoulders at right angles to the horse. The right leg moves forward on the off side of the horse during the movement.

§ 140. *Run, Hands on Croup, Back Straddle (Right Leg*

Leading), *and Half Right Circle with Right Leg to Ground.*
Run, place the hands on the croup and spring, pass the right
leg to the left in front of the left leg and carry it over the
horse from the near side to the off, raising the hands to let
it pass, replace the left hand on the croup and alight with
the shoulders at right angles to the horse. As you spring
you must cross the legs with the right leg in front, and turn
a little to the left ; the left leg moves forward on the off side
of the horse during the movement.

§ 141. *Run, Hands on Croup, Back Straddle* (*Left Leg
Leading*), *and Half Right Circle with Right Leg to Ground.*
Run, place the hands on the croup, and spring, pass the
right leg to the left behind the left leg, and carry it over
the horse from the near side to the off, raising the hands to
let it pass, replace the left hand on the croup, and alight
with the shoulders at right angles to the horse. As you
spring you must cross the legs, with the left leg in front,
and turn slightly to the right; the left leg moves forward
on the off side of the horse during the movement.

§ 142. You may do the exercises described in §§ 139–
141, and, after replacing the left hand, do a quarter or half
left turn before you alight; if you do a half left turn you
must let go with the left hand again, and place the right
hand on the horse as you alight.

§ 143 You may do exercises similar to those described
in §§ 139–141 with a bold spring, and alight opposite the
saddle or neck, or even beyond the neck ; but to get beyond
the neck is very difficult.

VAULTS.

§ 144. *Run, Hands on Croup, and Rear Vault Left to
Ground.* Run, place the hands on the croup, and spring,
carry both legs to the left, and then over the horse from

the near side to the off, raising the hands to let the legs pass, replace the left hand on the croup, and alight with the shoulders at right angles to the horse. The latter part of the movement is exactly like a rear vault left over the horse placed sideways.

§ 145. You may do the exercise described in the last paragraph, alighting with a quarter or half left turn. You may do similar exercises with the hands on the saddle or on the neck; the rear vault with the hands on the neck is rather difficult.

§ 146. *Run, Hands on Croup, and Flank Vault Left to Ground.* Begin as in the exercise described in § 144, but when you let go with the left hand, do a quarter right turn, hollow the back sharply, pass over the horse as if you were doing a flank vault over the horse placed sideways, and alight with your back to the horse.

§ 147. *Run, Hands on Croup, and Front Vault Left to Ground.* Begin as in the last exercise, but, instead of a quarter right turn, do a half right turn, pass over the horse as if you were doing a front vault over the horse placed sideways, and alight with the shoulders at right angles to the horse.

CIRCLES TO FRONT REST.

§ 148. The exercises described in §§ 139–141 and 144 may be done with a quarter left turn to a front rest on the off side of the horse. The exercise described in § 144, followed by the quarter left turn to the front rest, is, however, shortly described thus: "Run, hands on croup, carry the legs to the left, half right circle with both legs, and quarter left turn to front rest," the word "vault" being used only when the movement is made to the ground. In these movements, as you finish the half circle, you must turn sharply to the left, and place the hands on the near side of the horse. You must endeavour to reach the front rest with the back perfectly hollow, and the weight properly distributed between the hands and the thighs, so that you could do a vault, squat, or straddle, from the front rest without pause.

MOUNTS.

§ 149. *Run, Hands on Croup, Carry Legs to the Left, and Half Right Circle with Right Leg to Riding Seat on Croup.* Begin as if to do a rear vault left, as described in § 144, but, when the legs are over the horse, or rather sooner, straddle them, and alight in a riding seat. A similar movement may be done with the hands further forward on the croup to a riding seat in the saddle, or with the hands on the saddle or neck to a riding seat on the neck.

§ 150. *Run, Hands on Croup, Carry the Legs to the Left, and Half Right Circle with Left Leg, and Half Right Turn to Riding Seat on Croup Facing the Spring-board.* Begin as if to do a rear vault left, as explained in § 144, but, when the legs are on the near side of the horse, let the right thigh come in contact with the horse, let go with the left hand, do a half right turn, carrying the left leg over the horse, and rolling round on the right thigh, and come to the riding seat facing the spring-board. A similar movement may be done with the hands further forward on the croup to a riding seat on the saddle, or with the hands on the saddle or neck to a riding seat on the neck.

§ 151. *Run, Hands on Neck, and Straddle Mount to Riding Seat on Neck.* Run, spring, and place the hands on the neck, letting the legs swing up behind you with a hollow back, so that, when the hands reach the neck, you are in a free front lever exactly like that shown in Fig. 13, but, of course, with the body parallel to the horse, then straddle the

G

legs, and come to a riding seat on the neck just behind the hands. A similar mount may be done to the saddle with the hands on the neck just in front of the saddle, or to the croup with the hands on the saddle.

§ 152. *Run, Hands on Neck, and Back Straddle Mount to Riding Seat on Neck with Half Left Turn.* Begin as in the last exercise, then, the moment you reach the free front lever, do a half left turn, and come to the riding seat in the manner described in § 137. Similar exercises may be done to the riding seat on saddle or croup, placing the hands further back.

§ 153. *Run, Hands on Croup, and Straddle Mount to Riding Seat on Neck.* Run, place the hands on the croup, and spring, at the same moment press strongly from the hands and raise them, straddle the legs, fly through the air with the body upright, and the legs one on each side of the horse, and straddled as wide as possible, and alight in the riding seat on the neck without touching the horse again with the hands. This exercise requires considerable nerve; you may practise it at first to the riding seat on saddle, and, to make it easier, you may place the hands behind you on the horse as you reach the riding seat.

§ 154. *Run, Hands on Croup, and Back Straddle Mount to Riding Seat on Neck with Half Left Turn.* Run, place the hands on the croup, and spring, press strongly from the hands, and let go, at the same time cross the legs, as in the exercise described in § 140, and do a half left turn sharply, then fly through the air backwards, with the legs straddled and the body upright, and alight in the riding seat on the neck without touching the horse again with the hands. You may at first mount in this way to the saddle, and, to make the exercise easier, place the hands on the horse in front of you as you reach the riding seat.

§ 155. *Run, Hands on Croup, and Squat, and Straddle Mount to Riding Seat on Neck.* Run, place the hands on the croup, and spring, press strongly from the hands and let go, at the same time bend the knees, and carry the feet straight over the end of the croup with a movement similar to that made in squatting over the horse placed sideways, as explained in § 105, then shoot the legs out in front of you with a vigorous movement, and fly through the air with the body upright and the legs horizontal and straight, then straddle the legs, hollow the back sharply, and come to the riding seat on the neck. This movement is not at all easy; you may begin by mounting in this way to the saddle, placing the hands behind you as you reach the riding seat.

§ 156. *Run, Hands on Croup, and Straddle, and Front Shear Mount to Riding Seat on Neck with Half Left Turn.* Begin as if you meant to do a straddle mount, as described in § 153, but lean more back; then, the moment you let go, raise the legs above the horse, do a sharp half left turn, place the hands on the saddle, and close the legs, so that you reach a free front lever, straddle the legs, and alight in a riding seat on the neck facing the croup. As preliminary practice for this movement you may do the following exercise: Run, Hands on Croup, Half Right Circle with Left Leg with Quarter Left Turn to Front Rest, and Half Left Circle with Right Leg with Quarter Left Turn to Riding Seat Facing Croup. The movements made in doing the mount described above are almost identical with those made in this exercise.

§ 157. *Run, Hands on Croup, Carry Legs to the Left, and Front Shear Mount to Riding Seat on Saddle.* Begin as if to do a rear vault left, as explained in § 144, but, as the legs pass over the horse, do a sharp half left turn, and place the hands on the croup, so that you reach a free front lever, then straddle the legs, and come to a riding seat facing the croup. As preliminary practice for this mount you may do the following exercise : Run, Hands on Croup, Half Right Circle with Both Legs with Quarter Left Turn to Front Rest on Off Side of Horse, and Half Left Circle with Right Leg with Quarter Left Turn to Riding Seat. The movements made in doing the mount described above are almost identical with those made in this exercise.

§ 158. *Run, Hands on Croup, Back Straddle (Right Leg Leading), and Back Shear Mount to Riding Seat on Neck.* Begin as if you meant to do a back straddle mount with a half left turn, as explained in § 154, but lean more back, and turn as little to the left as you can, then let the legs come above the horse, turn back to the right, placing the left hand on the horse behind you, close the legs and straddle them again, carrying the left leg from the off side of the horse to the near, and the right leg from the near side of the horse to the off, passing the right leg over the left, and come to a riding seat on the neck with the back to the croup. As preliminary practice for this mount you may do the following exercise : Run, Hands on Croup, Back Straddle (Right Leg Leading), and Half Right Circle with Right Leg with Quarter Left Turn to Front Rest on Off Side of Horse, and Half Left Circle with Left Leg with Quarter Right Turn to Riding Seat. The movements made in doing the mount described above are almost identical with those made in this exercise.

DISMOUNTS.

§ 159. *Dismounts from Riding Seat on Neck Facing Neck—*

(i.) *Straddle to Ground.* Place the hands on the neck, throw the feet up behind you to a free front lever, then throw the head and shoulders sharply up from the hands, and straddle over the neck to the ground.

(ii.) *Squat to Ground.* Proceed as in the last exercise, but squat to the ground.

(iii.) *Back Shears to Ground with Half Left Turn.* Place the hands on the neck with the fingers pointing forwards, and then do back shears, as described in § 137, but press strongly from the right hand, and alight clear of the horse and facing it. As a preliminary exercise for this, you may practise back shears in the saddle, alighting . in front of your original position.

(iv.) *Back Shears to Ground without a Turn, Right Leg Leading.* Proceed as in the last exercise, but do not turn the shoulders at all, uncross the legs in the air, and alight with the back to the horse.

§ 160. *From Riding Seat on Neck Facing Croup, Front Shears with Half Left Turn to Ground.* Place the hands on the neck behind you, with the fingers well over the end of the neck, pointing downwards, the palms of the hands above the horse, and the thumbs separated from the fingers, and nearly vertical, so that so much of your weight as is supported on the hands rests almost entirely on the top joints of the thumbs. Sit close to the end of the neck, lean boldly back, and do front shears, as explained in § 138, very quickly, press strongly from the left hand, and alight with your back to the horse. This exercise seems almost impossible at first, but is not really very difficult. As a preliminary exercise, you may practise front shears in the saddle, alighting somewhat behind your original position.

LONG JUMPS.

§ 161. *Run, Hands on Neck, and Straddle Over.* Run, place the hands on the neck, and come to the free front lever, as in the straddle mount described in § 151, and then straddle over the neck to the ground. You must press very strongly from the hands as you straddle, and throw the head and shoulders well up, so that you keep your back almost hollow throughout the movement. Be very careful to keep the legs closed till you are fairly in the free front lever.

§ 162. *Run, Hands on Neck, and Squat Over.* Proceed exactly as in the last exercise, but squat over the neck to the ground instead of straddling. This exercise is not nearly so difficult as it looks.

§ 163. *Run, Hands on Neck, and Back Straddle Over with Half Left Turn.* Proceed as in the back straddle mount, described in § 152 ; but, instead of alighting in the riding seat, pass over the horse, and alight facing the neck. This movement is not easy to do well ; it is difficult to keep the legs straight, and very difficult to stand still when you alight.

§ 164. *Run, Hands on Croup, and Straddle Over.* Proceed as in the straddle mount with hands on croup, described in § 153, but fly completely over the horse, then close the legs and alight. This is not a difficult movement. You must be very careful to keep perfectly upright as you pass over the horse. If you let the shoulders come forward at all, the jump looks extremely clumsy, but, if properly done, it is a very pretty movement.

§ 165. *Run, Hands on Croup, and Straddle Over with Half Left Turn.* Begin as if you were going to do the straddle and front shear mount, described in § 156, but, when you have done your turn, press from the hands and pass over the horse without straddling the legs again, and alight facing it, with your hands on it. This is an easy jump, but it is a little difficult to keep exactly over the horse so that you alight quite straight beyond it.

§ 166. *Run, Hands on Croup, and Back Straddle Over with Half Left Turn.* Proceed as in the back straddle mount, described in § 154, but fly completely over the horse, and alight beyond it, facing the neck. This is not a difficult jump to do, but it is not easy to keep fairly over the middle of the horse so as to alight quite straight beyond it, and it is not at all easy to stand still when you alight.

§ 167. *Run, Hands on Croup, and Squat Over.* Begin as in the squat and straddle mount, described in § 155, but when you have shot the legs out in front of you, fly completely over the horse, feet first, and alight beyond it. This is far the most difficult of the long jumps, and wants considerable nerve and dash ; but it is very pretty, if it is well done.

§ 168. The long jumps described in §§ 161–167 are the principal exercises on the horse placed lengthways. In all the jumps the hands should be as near the end of the horse as possible. In jumps with the hands on the croup, you will find it advisable to place the spring-board back a yard or so from the horse, for if you jump from a point closer to the horse than that, you will not be able to place the hands at the extreme end of the horse.

In all jumps from the croup, your main object should be, after doing the exercise in good style, to jump as high and as far as you possibly can. In jumps with the hands on the neck, you should endeavour to show the free front lever quite distinctly, with the legs if anything higher than the head. In all straddle jumps you should straddle as wide as you can.

JUMPS OVER CROUP, RETURNING TO SPRING-BOARD.

§ 169. *Run, Straddle, and Front Shears over Croup to Ground.* Proceed as if to do a straddle and front shear mount to a riding seat on the croup, but when you straddle the legs again, straddle over the croup to the ground, so that you alight without the legs having touched the horse at all. ' This is not easy; you must take very little run, and lean well back as you begin, so that the shoulders remain over the spring-board throughout the movement, and you must do the movement very quickly.

§ 170. *Run, carry Legs to Left, and Front Shears over Croup to Ground.* Proceed as if to do the mount described in § 157, but when you straddle the legs, straddle over the croup to the ground again. The movement is a little more difficult than that described in the last paragraph, but is of the same character.

EXERCISES WITH HANDSTAND.

§ 171. *Reaching the Handstand.* You may reach a handstand on the horse without pommels with the shoulders at right angles to the horse in various ways.

(i.) From the riding seat, you may place the hands in front and lift to the handstand, either slowly, or quickly with a backward swing of the legs.

(ii.) From the riding seat, you may roll over backwards to the handstand. From the riding seat, swing the legs up sharply in front of you, bending at the waist, and, at the same time, let the head and shoulders drop back and come in contact with the horse, so that you lie on your back on the horse with the legs at right angles to the body; then, without pause, continue the movement, place the hands on the horse behind you, and hollow the back sharply, coming to the handstand. The movement resembles the roll over backwards to the double shoulderstand on the parallel bars, described in § 394. As you roll over, your weight is for an instant supported chiefly on the back of the head. The roll over backwards to the handstand is a difficult movement, and requires care at first, as you are very apt to fail in getting the hands placed on the horse; it is extremely difficult to retain the handstand after the movement.

(iii.) You may spring to the handstand in a manner similar to that described in § 128, and in this way you may reach a handstand on the croup, saddle, or neck.

§ 172. *Exercises from Handstand.* From the handstand you may do a variety of movements; some of which, however, are only possible from a handstand at one end of the horse. In discussing these movements, I shall assume that you have reached the handstand from a position facing the neck, so that in the handstand your back is towards the neck.

(i.) You may drop the feet, and either come to the riding seat or to the ground; from a handstand on the croup you may of course drop to the ground in this manner over the croup, alighting on the spring-board; from a handstand on the saddle or neck you must, in dropping to the ground, carry the feet a little to the right or left, and you will alight on one side of the horse, with a movement somewhat similar to a front vault behind one hand on the parallel bars (see § 426).

(ii.) From a handstand on the croup or saddle, you may roll over forwards to the riding-seat. When in the handstand, place the head on the horse just in front of the hands, bend at the waist, let the hips pass well forward, and let the back of the shoulders come in contact with the horse, then let go with the hands, continue the movement, and come to the riding seat. This movement is merely the reverse of the roll over backwards, described in the last paragraph. From a handstand on the neck just in front of the saddle, you may roll over forwards in a similar manner to the ground.

(iii.) From a handstand on the neck, just in front of the saddle, you may roll over to the ground with a movement similar to that last described, but, instead of placing the head on the horse, letting the head pass to the right or left, and placing one shoulder on the horse, so that before rolling over you come to a position similar to a shoulder-stand on the right shoulder on the left bar on the parallel bars (see § 405). This movement is called the "bear roll."

(iv.) From a handstand on the neck, you may do an overthrow to the ground, or squat or straddle over the neck to the ground. These movements are similar to those on the bar, described in §§ 249–253.

(v.) From a handstand with the shoulders at right angles to the horse, you may turn to a handstand with the shoulders parallel to the horse, and from that position do an over-throw, high front vault, squat or straddle to the ground, or turn back. These movements are similar to exercises in the handstand on the bar and parallel bars (see §§ 249–253, 401).

§ 173. The following are the most usual and characteristic exercises introducing handstands on the horse placed length-ways—

(i.) Run, Spring to Handstand with Hands on Neck, and Overthrow to Ground.

(ii.) From the Riding Seat on Neck, Swing up to Hand-stand, and Overthrow to Ground.

(iii.) Run, Spring to Handstand with Bent Arms with Hands on Neck, and Bear Roll to Ground.

(iv.) Run, Spring to Handstand on Croup or Saddle, and Roll Over Forwards to Riding Seat.

(v.) From the Riding Seat on Saddle facing Croup, Roll Over Backwards to Handstand, and Drop to Ground over Neck.

EXERCISES ON THE HORSE PLACED LENGTH-WAYS WITH POMMELS.

§ 174. The long jumps, the vaults to the ground with the hands on the croup, and several of the other exercises already described in Part II. of the present chapter, may of course be done on the horse placed lengthways, with pommels, exactly as if the pommels were not there; these exercises it is not necessary to describe further.

§ 175. You may do a straddle mount similar to that described in § 151, with the hands on the neck, the neck pommel, or the croup pommel, coming to a riding seat accordingly either on the neck, saddle, or croup. You may also do any one of these movements with a quarter left turn, placing the left hand behind you as you turn, and coming to a free side riding rest; the left hand must of course be placed on the neck pommel, croup pommel, or croup, according as you begin with the hands on the neck, neck pommel, or croup pommel. From the free side riding rest you may continue with any of the movements described in Part I. of the present chapter which begin from that position.

§ 176. You may do a series of back straddle mounts corresponding to the straddle mounts described in the last paragraph, and if you do these mounts with only a quarter turn, instead of a half turn, you may place one hand behind you and come to a free side riding rest, in a manner similar to that explained in the last paragraph.

§ 177. You may do a straddle mount with the hands on the croup, similar to that described in § 153, coming to a riding seat on the neck, saddle, or croup. As you do any of these movements you may do a quarter turn, and, instead of coming to a seat, place one hand on each side of you, and come to a free side riding rest on the neck, saddle, or croup, and continue as you please.

§ 178. You may do a back straddle mount with the hands on the croup similar to that described in § 154, coming to a riding seat on the neck, saddle, or croup. If you do such a movement with a quarter turn only, instead of a half turn, you may, instead of coming to a seat, place one hand on each side of you, and come to a free side riding rest on the neck, saddle, or croup.

§ 179. The exercises described in §§ 175–178, leading to a free side riding rest, are very easy to the croup, rather difficult to the saddle, and very difficult to the neck.

§ 180. You may do a straddle and front shear mount with the hands on the croup to a $_{.ri}d_{ing}$ seat in the saddle. After the turn in this mount you have, as has been explained in § 156, to place the hands behind you; now, instead of placing the hands on the croup, you may, if you do a half left turn, place the left hand on the croup, and the right hand on the croup pommel, and, instead of coming to a seat in the saddle, come to a rest, and continue as if you were doing a right feint. Perhaps a similar mount might be done to the neck, placing one hand on each pommel; but I have never seen it done.

§ 181. You may do exercises similar to those described in §§ 149, 150 with the hands on croup to a riding seat on croup, with the hands on croup pommel to a riding seat on saddle, or with hands on neck pommel to a riding seat on neck. You may also do these exercises with a quarter turn, and immediately place one hand beyond you, and come to a side riding rest. For example—

(i.) Run, Hands on Croup Pommel, Carry Legs to the Left, Half Right Circle with Right Leg with Quarter Right Turn, Place Left Hand on Neck Pommel, and continue as you please.

(ii.) Run, Hands on Croup Pommel, Carry Legs to the Left, Half Right Circle with Left Leg with Quarter Right Turn, Place Left Hand on Neck Pommel, and continue as you please.

In doing these exercises with the hands on either pommel it is generally advisable to take a grasp with the palm of the right hand upwards, so that when the movement is complete you have the ordinary grasp with that hand.

§ 182. Exercises similar to those described in the last paragraph may be done with a half circle with both legs coming to a free back rest.

§ 183. Front and back shears may be done in a manner similar to that described in §§ 137, 138, placing both hands on one pommel. In doing these movements you may, in the course of the shears, pass over the pommel, so that from a riding seat on the saddle you reach a riding seat on the neck, or croup, or *vice versâ.*

CHAPTER III.

THE HORIZONTAL BAR.

PART I.—*PRELIMINARY.*

§§ 184–187. Apparatus and General Definitions—§§ 188–190. The Grasp—§§ 191–199. Positions.

APPARATUS AND GENERAL DEFINITIONS.

§ 184. *Apparatus.* The horizontal bar should be about 7 ft. 6 in. long, and about $1\frac{3}{8}$ in. in diameter; it may be made of steel, either uncovered or covered with a thin veneer of wood or with leather. In my opinion a leather-covered bar is the pleasantest to work on. I believe that in Germany paper-covered bars are a good deal used, but I have never seen one of these.

§ 185. *Meaning of the Expressions " High Bar" and " Low Bar."* Exercises on the horizontal bar in general are most conveniently done either with the bar at such a height that you can hang from the bar at full length with the arms straight and the feet just clear of the ground when the toes are pointed, or with the bar at the height of the shoulders. A bar at the former height is called a "high bar," and a bar at the latter height is called a "low bar."

§ 186. *Side and Cross Positions.* Positions on the bar are divided into side and cross positions. All positions in which the shoulders are parallel to the bar are called "side" positions; all positions in which the shoulders are at right angles to the bar are called "cross" positions.

§ 187. *Meaning of the Expressions "In Front of Bar"
and "Behind Bar."* Suppose Fig. 14 represents the bar,
and that you are in any side position on the bar with the
upright marked C on your left. Then all points on the side
marked B of a vertical plane through the bar are said to
be in front of the bar, and all
points on the side marked A of
the same plane are said to be
behind the bar. If in the course
of an exercise you turn round,
points which were originally in
front of the bar will, after you
have turned, be behind the bar,
and *vice versâ.* It is accordingly
necessary, when using the expressions "in front of the bar"
and "behind the bar" in the

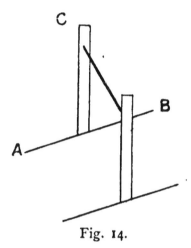

Fig. 14.

description of an exercise involving a turn, to state whether
the expressions are used with reference to the original. position
or to the ultimate position.

THE GRASP.

§ 188. *The Grasp in Side Positions.* If in any side
position you take hold of the bar with the left hand, with the
forefinger to the right, you have the ordinary grasp with
the left hand; similarly, if you take hold with the right
hand, with the forefinger to the left, you have the ordinary
grasp with the right hand. If in any side position you
take hold of the bar with the left hand, with the forefinger
to the left, the left hand being turned through a half left
turn from the ordinary grasp, you have the "reverse
grasp" with the left hand; similarly, if you take hold with
the right hand, with the forefinger to the right, the right

hand being turned through a half right turn from the ordinary grasp, you have the reverse grasp with the right hand. If in any side position you take hold of the bar with the left hand, with the forefinger to the left, the left hand being turned through a half right turn from the ordinary grasp, you have the "twisted grasp" with that hand, and a corresponding grasp with the right hand is the twisted grasp with that hand. If you have an ordinary grasp with one hand, and a reverse grasp with the other, you are said to have a "combined grasp."

If in any side position you have an ordinary grasp with one hand, and ordinary, reverse, or twisted grasp with the other, you cannot change the grasp with either hand without letting go the bar so long as you remain in the side position. If, however, you have the reverse grasp with both hands, you can in one position change to twisted grasp in a manner to be explained in § 216, while you remain in the side position, without letting go, and you can change in a similar manner from the twisted grasp to the reverse grasp, as is further explained in § 217. If from a side position you do a half turn, letting go with one hand, and come to a side position facing the other way, you will, of course, change the grasp of the hand which does not let go from the ordinary grasp to the reverse or twisted grasp, or *vice versâ*.

§ 189. *The Grasp in Cross Positions.* If in any cross position you grasp the bar with both hands with the palms of the hands towards each other and the wrists not crossed, you are said to have a "combined grasp." Any other grasp requires special description.

§ 190. *The Grasp Continued.* As a rule, if you grasp the bar with both hands, the clear distance between the hands should exceed the width of the hips by about an inch. The tendency of beginners is almost always to take the grasp much too wide. If, however, you have the twisted grasp with both hands, or with either hand, you will have to take a wider grasp.

Some gymnasts grasp the bar between the thumb and fingers, others with the fingers and thumb on the same side of the bar. Personally, I think the former method gives you a stronger and safer grip, especially in the reverse grasp. If, however, you have to use a very thick bar the latter method is certainly preferable, as a rule.

POSITIONS.

§ 191. *General Rules.* So far as nothing to the contrary appears, either expressly or by implication, in the description of any position on the bar, it is assumed—

(i.) That the position is to be a side, and not a cross, position.

(ii.) That the bar is to be grasped by both hands.

(iii.) That each hand is to have the ordinary grasp, and that the hands are to be at the usual distance apart.

(iv.) That the arms are to be straight and not crossed, and if the arms are directed to be bent, that they are, unless further directions are given, to be bent as much as possible.

(v.) That the legs are to be straight and closed, and are to hang vertically downwards, or as nearly vertically downwards as possible under the circumstances, and that, if the position of one leg is given, the other is to be straight and to hang vertically downwards, or as nearly vertically downwards as possible.

(vi.) That the body is to be upright, or as nearly upright as possible.

You must be careful to apply these rules only so far

H

as nothing to the contrary appears. If two of these rules in any particular position contradict each other, the earlier rule is to be followed.

§ 192. *Levers and Half Levers.* Positions in which the body is horizontal and the back hollow are called levers. If in any position the body is upright and the legs are horizontal, the legs are said to be in a half lever; and if, the body being upright, one leg is horizontal, that leg is said to be in a half lever.

§ 193. *Hanging Positions.* You may hang from the bar in a great variety of positions, supporting your weight either by the hands, or by one hand alone, or by the legs, or by one leg alone, or by the hands and legs, or in other ways, but in the absence of directions to the contrary, the word "hang," used either as a noun or as a verb, means hang by both hands with the forearms below the bar; and it is hanging positions of this kind alone which are discussed in the present paragraph.

Hangs are divided into "ordinary" and "back" hangs. If you jump up to a high bar, whatever grasp you take, you will be in an ordinary hang, and whatever position you assume, so long as you do not pass the feet through the arms and under the bar, and so long as you continue to hang at all, you remain in the ordinary hang (except that if the hands are wide apart in the twisted grasp you may come to a back hang with reversed grasp, as will be explained in § 217, without passing the feet through the hands). If, however, when in the ordinary hang, you pass the feet between the arms and under the bar, then, so long as you continue to hang without returning the feet between the arms, you are in the back hang (except that if you come to the back hang with reverse grasp with the hands wide apart you can, as will be explained in § 216, come to the ordinary hang with twisted grasp without returning the feet between the hands).

The intermediate positions, when one foot is passed through the arms and the other foot not, require no specific name, as the position is sufficiently indicated when the position of the feet or legs is given. If nothing to the contrary appears in the description of a hang, you are intended to be in an ordinary hang as distinguished from a back hang.

It may be pointed out that, in accordance with the rules given in § 191, the word "hang" used alone means hang with both hands in ordinary grasp, with the arms not crossed and straight, the body upright, the legs closed, straight, and pointing vertically downwards.

§ 194. *Leaning Hangs.* A leaning hang is a position in which you hang from the bar, supporting the weight partly by the hands or one hand and partly on some other limb or limbs.

§ 195. *Rests.* The word "rest" means that the weight is to be supported either entirely or partly on the hands, the forearms being above the bar and the feet not higher than the shoulders.

Rests are divided into "front rests," "back rests," "riding rests," and "rests astride one arm." If you stand facing a low bar, take hold of it and come to a rest on it, then, whatever grasp you take, and whatever position you assume, so long as you do not pass the feet through the arms and over the bar, and so long as you continue in a rest, you will remain in a "front rest." If, however, when in the front rest you pass the feet between the hands and over the bar, then, so long as you continue in a rest without returning the feet between the hands, you are in a "back rest." If nothing to the contrary appears in the description of a rest, you are intended to be in a front rest as distinguished from a back rest.

"Rest," without further explanation, means, in accordance with the rules given, a position just like a front rest on the horse (see § 23). Similarly, "back rest," without further explanation, means a position just like a back rest on the horse (see § 23). The intermediate position between a front and back rest, in which one leg has been passed between the hands and the other not, is called a "riding rest" if the legs are astride the bar, and a "rest astride one arm," if both legs are in front of the bar with one hand between them. It may be pointed out that, in accordance with the rules given in § 191, "riding rest," without further explanation, means a position just like a side riding rest on the horse (see § 23), and "rest astride one arm," without further explanation, means a position similar to a rest astride one arm on the horse (see § 65), but with the feet considerably lower. If from a side seat on the bar (see § 197) you grasp the bar between the legs and raise most of the weight on the arms, the position you reach is called the "straddle rest."

§ 196. *Free Rests.* The word "free" in the description of a rest means that the legs are not to touch the bar; most free rests are only momentary positions, that is to say, you cannot remain in them. "Free rest," "free back rest," and "free riding rest," mean respectively positions similar to the free front rest, the free back rest, and the free side riding rest, on the horse.

§ 197. *Seats.* The expressions "side seat" and "cross seat" have the same meaning as in the case of the horse; the phrase "riding seat" has the same meaning as the phrase "side riding seat" in the case of the horse, and the phrase "cross riding seat" has the same meaning as the phrase "riding seat" in the case of the horse (see § 22). It should be pointed out that the same position may often be described either as a seat with the hands on the bar or as a rest. Sometimes one method of description is more convenient, and sometimes the other.

§ 198. *Handstands.* If you support the body on the hands above the bar, with the body vertical and the head downwards, you are said to be in a handstand. Handstands on the parallel bars are shown in Figs. 20, 22.

§ 199. There are positions on the bar which do not fall into the various categories hitherto dealt with, for example, hanging positions from the knees or feet, but these may be left for the present.

The system upon which positions on the bar are described may seem somewhat complex at first; but, in practice, you will find it very simple. It is so arranged that all positions of frequent occurrence may be very shortly described. A few positions, which it would be troublesome to describe in accordance with the system, have recognized short names, which tends further to shorten the language. These names will be given in the course of the chapter.

PART II.—*SLOW EXERCISES.*

§§ 200-217. Exercises in the Hang—§§ 218-224. Exercises in the Rest—§§ 225-240. Exercises leading from Hang to Rest, and *vice versâ*—§ 241. Exercises introducing Handstands and Levers above the Bar.

EXERCISES IN THE HANG.

§ 200. Slow exercises, which begin from a hang, should be practised on a high bar. At the beginning of the exercise you must of course jump to the hang. You should be careful to jump from exactly below the bar, otherwise you will have a slight swing when you reach the hang, and you will have to stop this before you continue. Be careful also to pause an instant in the hang with perfectly straight arms before you proceed with your exercise, unless of course you are told to jump to a hang with bent arms.

§ 201. *Hang, Rise to Bent Arm Hang, Sink to Straight Arm Hang.* Hang with straight arms, rise to the bent arm hang by bending the arms slowly, then let the arms slowly unbend again and return to the straight arm hang. Be careful throughout the whole exercise to keep the back quite hollow; when in the bent arm hang the bar should be opposite the chest, the head up, with the chin pressed back. This exercise often goes by the name of pulling up to the chin, and beginners are apt, in an effort to do it many times in succession, to let the body bend at the waist, and to rise just high enough to poke the chin over the bar; it is better to be content to do the movement comparatively few times in proper style. This exercise may be done with ordinary, reverse, or combined grasp, also with one hand in twisted grasp and the other hand in ordinary or reverse grasp. I doubt its being possible with both hands in twisted grasp.

§ 202. *Hang, Raise Legs, or One Leg, to Half Lever.* Hang, raise the legs, or one leg, to a horizontal position, keeping the legs and arms straight; this may be done with all the different grasps.

§ 203. *Hang, Raise Feet to Bar.* Hang, raise the legs, keeping the arms and legs perfectly straight until the feet almost touch the bar. This is a movement of fundamental importance, but requires considerable strength, and you must not be disappointed if it takes you a long time to learn. I know no exercise which seems more completely impossible when you first try it. You may at first bend the knees, straightening them when the feet reach the bar. If you cannot raise the feet to the bar even with bent knees, you may bend the arms also at the beginning of the movement, and then straighten them again. You may also, when you make some progress with the exercise, raise the feet to the bar with bent knees, and then straighten the legs, and let them sink slowly from the bar till you come to the hang with straight arms. You may consider that you do the exercise well if you can raise the feet with a perfectly even movement, and take over ten seconds to do the whole movement. Do not imagine that you take over that time merely because the exercise seems to take a long time, but get a friend with a watch to time you. Of course it is easy enough to take much longer, if you begin exceedingly slowly, and then hurry when you reach the difficult part; but the first essential is to do the movement in perfectly even time, so that the feet always move through an equal distance in an equal time. You may do this exercise with all the different grasps; with a twisted grasp it is difficult.

§ 204. *Hang, Raise Feet to Bar, Hollow the Back, bringing Thighs to Bar.* Hang, and raise the feet to the bar, then hollow the back so that you hang head downwards, with the thighs almost touching the bar. In this position the body and legs will not be vertical, but the feet will be rather in front of the bar, and the head behind it; it is not easy to retain this position at first. You may do this exercise with all the different grasps; with a twisted grasp it is very difficult.

§ 205. *Hang, with Hollow Back and Thighs to Bar, Sink to Front Lever.* From the hang mentioned, let the legs and body sink, keeping the back hollow, until the body

and legs are perfectly horizontal.   The front lever, which is
shown in Fig. 15, is extremely difficult to retain, and requires,

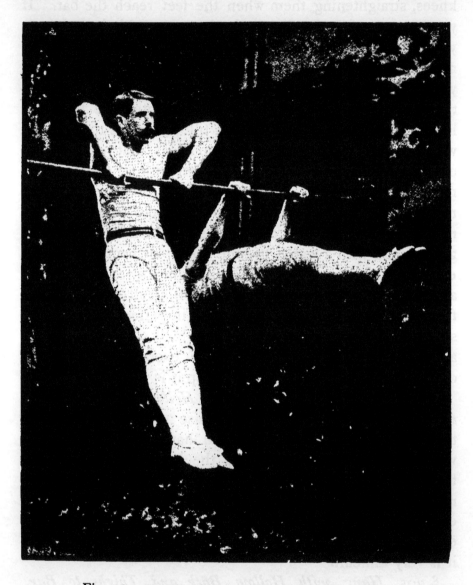

Fig. 15.—FRONT LEVER AND BENT ARM REST.

except in the case of men very ill-developed in the lower
limbs, quite exceptional strength.   You may at first

attempt it with one knee bent and one foot hooked behind the knee of the other leg. The front lever can be done with ordinary, reverse, or combined grasp. I have never seen it done with either hand in twisted grasp, but I suppose it is possible. With both hands in a twisted grasp it would be a marvellous exhibition of strength. You will find it impossible at first to tell for yourself whether you are horizontal or not, and you will have to get some one to tell you; in course of time, however, you will learn to recognize the position for yourself.

§ 206. You may rise with a hollow back from the hang to the front lever, or from a front lever to a hang hollow back with thighs to the bar, and you may sink from a front lever to a hang. You may also do a front lever with bent arms, and rise and sink between a front lever with straight arms and a front lever with bent arms. You may do a front lever with combined grasp with the arms crossed, and then let the body rotate in a horizontal plane so that you pass through a front lever in the cross hang, and come to a front lever with the arms uncrossed, and you may do a similar rotation from a front lever with the arms uncrossed to a front lever with crossed arms. All these exercises are of extreme difficulty.

§ 207. *Hang, Raise Feet to Bar, Pass Feet between Arms to Back Hang with Heels to Bar, Sink to Back Hang.* Hang and raise the feet to the bar, as described in § 203, then bend the knees, pass the feet between the arms under the bar, straighten the knees again, bringing the heels close to the bar, then let the feet sink behind the bar till the legs hang vertically downwards, then let the body sink as low as you can, till you hang nearly upright.

Some men can pass the feet between the arms without bending the knees; but I doubt if any grown man can learn to do this unless he can very nearly do it naturally; however, if you are quite young, or naturally so supple that you can nearly accomplish this movement, it is worth while to devote a good deal of practice to it, as, once accomplished, it will enable you to do a number of exercises on the bar in a style which most men cannot approach. On the other hand, many men have great difficulty in getting the feet between the arms at all, almost all men can, however, learn to do it with practice; if you find it very difficult, you may at first cross the feet, which will give you a little more room. The exercise described above may be done with ordinary, reverse, or combined grasp, or with one hand in twisted grasp and the other in ordinary or reverse grasp, and it is possible with both hands in twisted grasp, but with that grasp it requires exceptional suppleness.

§ 208. *From the Back Hang, Raise Feet to Bar, Pass Legs between Arms to Ordinary Hang with Feet to Bar.* This is merely the reverse of the last part of the exercise described in the last paragraph; it is not difficult. You may try it at first with bent knees. It is a little easier to bring the feet between the arms with the legs straight, passing from the back hang to the ordinary hang, than in the other direction. This exercise may be done with the same variety of grasp as that described in the last paragraph.

§ 209. *From the Back Hang, Heels to Bar, Hollow the Back to Back Hang with Hollow Back and Thighs to Bar.* Come to the back hang with heels to the bar, then hollow the back till you are hanging head downwards, with the back hollow and the back of the thighs almost touching the bar. This position is not difficult to retain; in it you must keep the head well back. This exercise may be done with the same variety of grasp as those described in the last two paragraphs.

§ 210. *From the Back Hang with Hollow Back and Thighs to Bars, Sink to Back Lever.* Come to the position described in the last paragraph, then let the legs and body sink behind the bar, keeping the back hollow, until the body and legs are horizontal. The back lever is difficult to retain ; but not nearly so difficult as the front lever. You may try it at first with bent knees, or one knee bent. You will find it difficult at first to tell for yourself whether you are horizontal in this position, and you must get some one to tell you, until you learn to recognize the position for yourself. The back lever may be done with ordinary, reverse, or combined grasp, or with one hand in twisted grasp and the other hand in ordinary or reverse grasp ; it is possible with both hands in twisted grasp, but is extremely difficult.

§ 211. You may rise from the back hang to the back lever, hollowing the back gradually, and you may rise from the back lever to the back hang with hollow back and thighs to bar, and you may sink from a back lever to the back hang.

§ 212. *From the Back Lever, Quarter Left Turn to Side Lever on Right Arm.* Come to the back lever, then do a quarter left turn, at the same time bending the right arm, and getting the whole weight on to it, so that you come to a horizontal position with the right flank towards the ground and with the right forearm passing across the hollow of the back, and in contact with it. In this position you may let go with the left hand coming to a "side lever on the right arm alone," in which position the left arm may be held straight in front of the head in a straight line with the legs and body, or placed close to the left side. The side lever on the right arm alone is shown in Fig. 16 ; the left arm should, however, be more in a straight line with the body than in **the** figure. You may do a side lever on the. right arm with the right hand in reverse grasp,

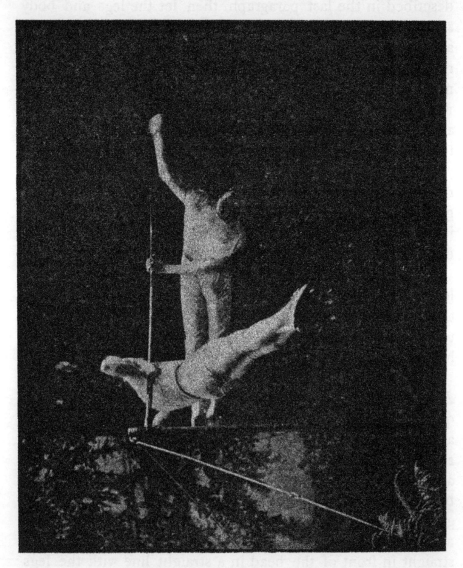

Fig. 16.—SIDE LEVER ON RIGHT ARM ALONE AND CROSS BENT ARM REST ON RIGHT ARM ALONE.

but, in that case, you will not be able to keep the body

at right angles to the bar; the feet will pass to the right and the shoulders to the left, so that your body will be parallel to the bar. You may also do a side lever on the right arm with the right hand in twisted grasp; but in that case your legs will pass to the left and the shoulders to the right, so that your body will be parallel to the bar. You may of course do a side lever on the right arm with the left hand in ordinary, reverse, or twisted grasp. You may reach the side lever on the right arm from the back hang with hollow back and thighs to the bar, without first coming to the back lever, by letting the feet pass to the right, and then sinking the feet and raising the shoulders, keeping the right forearm close to the back all the time. You may also reach the side lever on one arm from the back hang with body and legs vertical, raising the feet with a hollow back, and turning to the left simultaneously.

§ 213. In the side lever on the right arm alone, you may let the body revolve in a horizontal plane, about the right forearm as an axis. In this manner you can revolve altogether through a little more than two right angles, coming from a position in which your body is nearly parallel to the bar, with the feet to the left, and a little behind the bar, to a position in which your body is nearly parallel to the bar, with the feet to the right, and a little behind the bar, or *vice versâ*. Of course you may do exercises involving a revolution of this kind of less extent.

The following exercises introduce movements of this kind—

(i.) From a back lever with reverse grasp, turn to side lever on the right arm, letting the feet pass to the right, let go with the left hand, let the body revolve through a right angle until the body is at right angles to the bar (the head is now behind the bar, reckoning from your original position), take hold of the bar with the left hand with ordinary grasp (placing the hand on the bar at a point to the right of right hand, reckoning from your original position), and quarter right turn to back lever with ordinary grasp.

(ii.) From the back hang, with hollow back and thighs to bar, and right hand in twisted grasp, sink to side lever on the right arm, letting the feet pass to the left, let go with the left hand, let the body revolve through a little more than two right angles, place the left hand on the bar in its original position, with reverse grasp, and quarter right turn, letting the feet move to the left, and coming to back lever with reverse grasp.

§ 214. I have seen acrobats raise the body with a sort of twist from the straight arm hang on one arm to the side lever on that arm alone; but I have never seen an amateur do it. It is not very difficult to sink from the side lever on one arm to the straight arm hang on that arm, letting the body gradually untwist and the feet sink.

§ 215. It is possible to come to a side lever on the right arm with the arm in front of the body, and in that position you may let go with the left hand, coming to a side lever on the right arm alone with the arm in front of the body. You may reach this side lever from the front lever with a quarter right turn, or you may reach the lever direct from the hang, or from the hang with the feet or thighs to the bar. · The side lever on the right arm with the arm in front of the body is, however, a very ungainly position, as it is impossible to keep the back hollow. You may of course, reach this lever with the right hand in various grasps, and in the lever you may pivot about the right forearm as an axis, in a manner similar to that described in § 213.

§ 216. *From the Back Hang with Reverse Grasp and Hands Wide Apart, Dislocate to Ordinary Hang with Twisted Grasp.* Come to the back hang with a reverse grasp with the hands wide apart, let the shoulders turn in their sockets, and come to the ordinary hang with twisted grasp. This movement is peculiar and difficult to describe. If you take a long stick and hold it behind your back with a reverse grasp, and then pass it over your head and down in front of the body you will have done this movement with the shoulders, and you will find that you have a twisted grasp of the stick.

§ 217. *From the Ordinary Hang with Twisted Grasp and Hands Wide Apart, Dislocate to Back Hang with Reverse Grasp.* Come to the hang with twisted grasp with the hands wide apart, raise the hips a little and let the shoulders turn in their sockets, coming to the back hang with reverse grasp. This exercise is simply the reverse of that described in the last paragraph.

EXERCISES IN REST.

§ 218. Slow exercises in the rest may be conveniently practised at first on a low bar, on which, of course, you can easily spring into the rest. The twisted grasp is of no practical use in the rest.

§ 219. *From Rest, Sink to Bent Arm Rest and Rise to Rest.* From the rest, let the weight sink by bending the arms, at the same time letting the legs come forward under the bar, until the arms are as much bent as possible; straighten the arms and return to the rest. The bent arm rest is shown in Fig. 15. You must be careful to keep the head up in this position. The exercise may be done with ordinary, reverse, or combined grasp.

§ 220. *From Back Rest, Sink to Back Rest with Bent Arms and Rise to Back Rest.* From the back rest, let the weight sink by bending the arms, keeping the back hollow, until the arms are as much bent as possible, then straighten the arms and return to the back rest. This is extremely difficult to do really slowly; it is almost necessary to descend with a slight swing and rise with the return swing; done in this manner it is very easy; it may be done with ordinary, reverse, or combined grasp.

§ 221. *From Rest, Sink to Bent Arm Rest, Quarter Left Turn, Letting go Left Hand, to Cross Bent Arm Rest on Right Arm Alone.* Sink from the rest to the bent arm rest, then turn to the left, bringing the right arm-pit almost in contact with the bar, let go with the left hand and hold the left arm out horizontally. In this position, which is shown in Fig. 16, the back should be hollow. It is not a difficult position to retain.

§ 222. *From Cross Bent Arm Rest on Right Arm Alone, Quarter Left Turn to Back Rest with Bent Arms.* From the cross bent arm rest on the right arm alone, turn to the left and place the left hand on the bar so that you are in the back rest with bent arms, you will, of course, now have a reverse grasp with the right hand, with the left hand you may take either ordinary or reverse grasp. This movement is difficult after coming to a stationary position in the cross bent arm rest on the right arm alone, but if you turn into that rest from the bent arm rest on both arms, and continue turning without a pause, it is comparatively easy.

§ 223. *From Back Rest with Bent Arms with Right Hand Reversed, Half Right Turn to Cross Bent Arm Rest on Right Arm Alone.* This requires no further description, it is merely the reverse of the exercise described in the last paragraph.

§ 224. *From Back Rest with Bent Arms, Half Right Turn to Cross Bent Arm Rest on Right Arm Alone with Back of Hand towards Body.* This is exactly like the exercise described in the last paragraph, except that you start from a back rest with bent arms with the ordinary grasp ; the cross bent arm rest on the right arm alone with the back of the hand to the body, which you reach in this way, is extremely difficult to retain. You may, of course, from that rest turn to the left and come to the back rest with bent arms with the right hand in ordinary grasp.

EXERCISES LEADING FROM HANG TO REST, AND VICE VERSÂ.

§ 225. *From the Bent Arm Hang, Raise Right Elbow above Bar.* In the bent arm hang, shift most of the weight on to the left arm and raise the right elbow above the bar, so that you are in the bent arm hang from the left hand, and bent arm rest on the right arm. You may continue in various ways ; you may let go with the left hand and come to the cross bent arm rest on the right arm alone, or you may shift the weight on to the right arm and raise the left elbow above the bar, thus coming to a bent arm rest on both arms. For these exercises, you must begin with the right hand in ordinary grasp, but the left may have either ordinary or reverse grasp.

§ 226. *Hang and Slow Rise to Rest.* Hang and rise to bent arm hang, then let the feet come under the bar by bending at the waist, raise the elbows gradually until you come to the bent arm rest ; then rise to the rest. In order to do this exercise you must take a peculiar grip of the bar. To learn this grip you may proceed as follows : stand facing the bar with the bar about your own height, place the hands over the bar keeping them open, bend the wrists till your forearms are nearly vertical, and the hands nearly at right angles to them so that the wrists rest against the bar, then turn the hands inwards and grasp the bar with the ordinary grasp but without letting the wrists slip at all, so that the bar is now grasped in the hands but the back of the hands are above the bar and the bar touches the outside of the wrists, and you have the proper grip for a slow rise. You will at first find it extremely difficult to retain this grip with the arms perfectly straight. You may accordingly at first begin a slow rise with the arms slightly bent. The slow rise is not easy; if you make the movement even from the hang to the rest and take over twelve seconds to do it, you may consider that you do it well. If you come to the hang after some preceding movement, which does not allow of your having the grip explained, and wish to continue with a slow rise, you must shift the hands to this grip with a jerk as you are rising to the bent arm hang. The exercises described in the last paragraph are good practice for the slow rise.

§ 227. *From the Rest, Sink to Hang.* From the rest, sink to bent arm rest, and continue sinking till you come to the hang, letting the elbows pass gradually down behind the bar; this is simply the reverse of the last exercise. If you propose to do the slow rise after this exercise, you must, as the elbows sink past the bar, turn the wrists slightly outwards and keep the wrists above the bar, so that when you come to the hang you have the proper grip for a slow rise. On the other hand, if you intend to continue in any other manner, you must let the grip slip gradually as you descend.

§ 228. *Hang with Right Hand in Reverse Grasp, Rise to Bent Arm Rest, and Raise Right Elbow above Bar with Three Quarter Left Turn in Course of Movement.* Hang with combined grasp, right hand reversed, bend the elbows, at the same time turning to the left so that, as you rise, the head passes under the bar; when you come to the bent arm hang, continue turning and raise the right elbow above the bar, if you then let go with the left hand you will be in a cross bent arm rest on the right arm alone in front of the

bar (reckoning from your original position). In this movement you must be careful to move quite steadily without
any pause or jerk ; the secret of the movement is to turn
the head well over the left shoulder at first and keep it there
throughout the movement. The movement is made easier
by taking the grasp with the hands rather close to each
other.

§ 229. Several exercises may be done somewhat similar
to that described in the last paragraph. You may do an
exactly similar movement beginning with the arms crossed.
Again, you may begin from a cross bent arm rest on the left
arm alone, then take hold of the bar with the right hand in
reverse grasp on either side of the left hand with the elbow
below the bar, and then let the left elbow sink below the
bar, pass under the bar and raise the right elbow above it
on the other side with a complete left turn in the course of
the movement.

§ 230. Exercises similar to those described in the last
two paragraphs may be done with both hands in ordinary
grasp ; when you rise above the bar in these exercises, you
will come to the cross bent arm rest on the right arm with
the back of the hand to the body described in § 224. These
movements are extremely difficult, the easiest of them is
a rise from a hang with the arms crossed.

§ 231. *Hang, Slow Circle to Rest.* Hang and raise the
feet to the bar, as explained in § 203 ; then bend the arms
keeping the feet still pointing upwards so that the thighs
come opposite the bar, then pass the legs over the bar, at
the same time letting the stomach come in contact with it,
and slowly hollow the back so that you come to the
rest. In the description of this exercise I have used
the phrase "slow circle," to mean the whole movement from
the hang ; however it is often used to mean the last part

of the movement, from the hang with feet to the bar, alone.
The slow circle can be done with all the different grasps;
if you have a twisted grasp with either hand, you must let
go with that hand as you pass over the bar and take a fresh
grasp, and if you have twisted grasp with both hands you
must let go with both hands. The slow circle is an important exercise; as will appear later, similar exercises may be
done quickly. As preliminary practice for all these exercises,
you may, on a low bar, try to do a movement similar to the
slow circle, starting from the ground with a jump, bending
the arms and doing the movement quickly, being careful,
however, always to keep the legs straight. When you can
do this you may try it placing the bar a little higher, and
then higher still, until you can do it on a high bar quickly;
you may then try to do it more and more slowly and
with less and less bend of the arms before the feet come to
the bar.

§ 232. *From the Rest, Slow Roll Over Forwards to Hang.*
From the rest, let the head and shoulders sink in front of
the bar till you come to a leaning hang on the thighs with
bent arms, then raise the thighs from the bar and let the
arms straighten, coming to a hang with feet to the bar, then
let the legs sink slowly to the hang. This exercise is merely
the reverse of the slow circle.

§ 233. *Hang with Right Hand Reversed, and Slow Circle
to Side Seat outside Left Hand.* From the hang mentioned,
proceed as if to do a slow circle, as described in § 231; as
the legs pass over the bar move them a little to the left and
let the left thigh come in contact with the bar, outside the
left hand, then let the head and shoulders pass to the right
and raise the right elbow above the bar, at the same time
rolling round on the left thigh, continue the movement,
gradually straightening the right arm and bringing the left

elbow above the bar, then let go with the right hand and you will find yourself in a side seat on the bar with the left hand reversed. The result of the movement is the same as if you had done a slow circle to the rest and then a half right turn to the side seat outside the left hand.

§ 234. *From Back Hang with Hollow Back and Thighs to Bar, Slow Circle Behind Bar to Back Rest.* Hang in the back hang with the thighs to the bar, as explained in § 209, bend the arms, still keeping the back hollow and the feet pointing upwards; let the legs pass over the bar and let the back come in contact with it, at the same time letting the weight pass over the bar, raising the head and dropping the feet till you come to the back rest. This movement is very easy for thin men, and very difficult for stoutly made men; it may be done with ordinary, combined, or reverse grasp; with reverse grasp, however, almost all men find it difficult. I should doubt its being possible with a twisted grasp. Beginners are apt, in doing the slow circle behind the bar, to let the legs bend and separate quite unconsciously, you must be careful to avoid this.

§ 235. From the side lever on the right arm alone you may place the left hand on bar with the elbow above it. This exercise admits of considerable variety; you may come to the lever in question in several positions as explained in § 212, and then place the left hand on the bar without changing the position of the body; or from any one of these positions you may revolve about the right forearm to a greater or less extent, as explained in § 213, and then place the left hand on the bar. For example, if you come to the back lever with reverse grasp and then turn to the side lever on the right arm alone, you may place the left hand on the bar in four ways, namely (reckoning always from your original position as explained in § 187) ·

(i.) Without revolving at all, behind the bar to the original left of the right hand.

(ii.) After a slight revolution, behind the bar to the original right of the right hand.

(iii.) After a further revolution, in front of the bar to the original right of the right hand.

(iv.) After a still further revolution, in front of the bar to the original left of the right hand.

After placing the left hand on the bar you may let go with the right hand and come to the cross bent arm rest on the left arm alone, or, in some positions, you may raise the right elbow above the bar and come to the back rest with bent arms, as in the exercises described in the next paragraph.

§ 236. *From the Side Lever on Right Arm Retaining Grasp of Left Hand, Raise Left Elbow above Bar, and then Shift Right Elbow above Bar, coming to Back Rest with Bent Arms.* The first part of this exercise is very like some of the movements described in the last paragraph, but the left arm is shifted from the hang to the rest without letting go; then the weight is shifted on to the left arm and the right elbow raised. The exercise may be done with ordinary, reverse, or combined grasp with either hand reversed. It is easiest with the right hand in ordinary grasp and the left hand in reverse grasp.

§ 237. *From the Back Rest with Bent Arms, Let Right Elbow Sink in Front of Bar and turn to Side Lever on Right Arm.* This is simply the reverse of the exercise described in the last paragraph, and may be done with the same variety of grasp.

§ 238. *From the Back Rest with Reverse Grasp and Bent Arms, Sink to Back Lever and Sink to Back Hang.* From the back rest with reverse grasp and bent arms, gradually straighten the arms letting the shoulders move forward, and at the same time raising the feet behind the bar, then let the elbows sink below the bar and come to a back lever, then let the legs sink to the back hang.

§ 239. It is, I believe, possible to do a slow rise from the back hang with reverse grasp to the back rest, but I have never seen it done; it is, of course, merely the reverse of the exercise described in the last paragraph.

§ 240. Exercises similar to those described in §§ 235, 236, may be done from the side lever on the right arm with the arm in front of the body described in § 215, leading to a cross bent arm rest on the left arm alone, or to a bent arm rest; these exercises are, however, very inelegant.

EXERCISES INTRODUCING HANDSTANDS AND LEVERS ABOVE THE BAR.

§ 241. A great number of slow exercises may be done on the bar leading from the rest to a handstand or a lever in the rest, or to elbow levers, or from these positions to the rest. Some of these exercises are actually described in Chapter IV. (see §§ 417–420). The others are so similar to exercises described in that chapter (see §§ 373, 387, 389, 390, 392, 398, 402, 411, 412) that it is unnecessary to deal with them here.

PART III.—QUICK EXERCISES.

§§ 242–247. Vaults, Leg Circles, Feints, Shears, Squatting and Straddling Movements—§§ 248–253. Exercises introducing Handstands—§§ 254–277. Knee, Mill, and Seat Circles—§§ 278–293. Swinging—§§ 294–298. Upstarts—§ 299. Swing and Knee Seat and Mill Circles—§§ 300–304. Clear Circle, Short Circle, Front

Circle, and Hand Circle—§§ 305-309. Back-Up—§§ 310-312.   Long Circles and Half Long Circles— §§ 313-324.   Combination of Exercises—§§ 325-326. Changing Grasp—§§ 327-340.   Turns, Giant Back- Up, etc.—§§ 341-345.   Exercises in Back Hang— §§ 346-352.   Miscellaneous Exercises.

VAULTS, LEG CIRCLES, ETC.

§ 242. You may do vaults, circles with the legs, feints, shears, and straddling and squatting movements on the bar very much in the same way as on the horse, and these exercises may most of them be done with ordinary, reverse, or combined grasp; they may be begun from a front or back rest, or from a riding rest according to the nature of the movement.   In combination with other movements they may, of course, many of them also be begun from the corresponding free rests without pause.   Such of the exercises as may be begun from a front rest may also on a low bar be begun from the ground.   How far it would be possible to carry these movements it is difficult to say, there seems to be no physical impossibility about doing on the bar almost any of the circling and vaulting exercises which can be done on the horse; practically, however, you will find that all but the very simplest exercises of this nature are of almost insurmountable difficulty.   Such of these exercises as are usually accomplished, are shortly discussed in the next few paragraphs.

§ 243. *Vaults.* On a high bar, you are practically confined to flank and front vaults; you must, of course, in both these vaults, let go altogether as you are descending. The great difficulty about them is to alight steadily. On a low bar you may do a rear or screw vault besides. In doing a screw vault right on the bar, you do the same turn as in a screw vault right on the horse ; but, the moment you start, let go with the *left* hand and pass over the bar with the whole weight on the right arm, and descend, still holding with the right hand. It is, of course, impossible to do this with the right hand in reverse grasp. In doing flank, front, or screw vaults from the rest, throw the legs back a few inches, let the arms bend slightly, and drop on to the lower part of the stomach, let the legs swing under the bar, and then, as they swing back again, spring from the stomach and do the vault, throwing the weight boldly over the bar as you begin the vault. In the rear vault from the rest, however, start directly from the rest without sinking to the rest on the stomach first.

§ 244. *Feints.* The ordinary feint is the only feint which you will find it practically possible to do.

§ 245. *Leg Circles and Shears.* Complete circles from the rest with one leg are difficult, and with both legs extremely difficult; but the half circles from the rest with one leg, or both legs, are fairly easy and must be thoroughly mastered. In beginning these exercises from the rest, you must start direct from the rest without sinking on to the stomach. The chief difficulty in doing these half circles, is to retain the balance when the half circle is complete so that you can remain in the side riding rest or back rest, as the case may be. The half circle with both legs is the most difficult, you must keep the hips close to the arm which is not raised, carry the legs only just over the bar, and let them sink low in front of the bar so that when you reach the back rest your back is almost hollow; if you keep the legs too high so that the thighs come in contact with the bar, it is almost impossible to make sure of not over-balancing. Half circles from the back rest with one leg are not difficult, and complete circles with one leg are not very difficult. The half circle with both legs is difficult, but can be done;

you should be able to do this to a free rest, ready to continue with swinging exercises. A complete circle with both legs from the back rest, I have never seen accomplished. The word "circle," is used not only for these exercises, but also as the word has been already used in §§ 231, 234, to describe movements of another nature altogether. In any case in which confusion could arise, it is advisable to describe the exercises dealt with in this paragraph as "leg circles." Front and back shears can be done on the bar, but are not easy.

§ 246. *Squatting and Straddling Movements.* Squatting and straddling exercises, like those on the horse, can be done on the bar, and require little fresh explanation. If you intend to squat right over the bar from the rest, with a movement like that explained in § 105 (i.), you should first sink on to the stomach, as explained in § 243. If you intend to come to the back rest, or to squat with one leg, you should start direct from rest. The squat backwards with both legs is decidedly difficult. In all squatting exercises on the bar in which you are going to pass the legs between the arms, you must bring the knees well up to the chest. You may straddle over the bar either to the ground, the back rest, or the straddle rest. If you start from the rest and intend to come to the ground, sink on to the stomach to start, as explained above. If you intend to come to the back rest, bring the legs right over the bar and come to a straddle rest before you let go.

§ 247. Exercises may be done on the bar somewhat similar to those on the horse in which a circle over the saddle is followed by a movement over the neck or croup ; but these exercises will be more conveniently discussed hereafter ; they are all difficult.

EXERCISES INTRODUCING HANDSTANDS.

§ 248. *From the Rest, Throw up to Handstand.* From the rest, sink on to the stomach and then throw the legs back through the free rest till the legs come right above your head, and you are in a handstand. You may come to the handstand with either bent arms or straight arms, and with ordinary, combined, or reverse grasp. The handstand is a very difficult position to retain on a thin bar, but it is a position from which many exercises may be done, if you reach it momentarily.

§ 249. *From the Handstand, Overthrow to Ground.* In the handstand, let the weight pass in front of the bar, and, the moment you are overbalanced, bring the head forward (that is to say, bring the chin in to the breast), push strongly from the arms, let go and alight in front of the bar. After you let go you do a portion of a front somersault in the air. This overthrow is easy with bent arms, with straight arms it is rather difficult; it may be done with ordinary, combined, or reverse grasp. On a high bar you must be careful not to push too hard as you let go, or you will be apt to fall on your face. The expression "overthrow," is sometimes used to include throwing up to the handstand.

§ 250. *From the Handstand, Overthrow and Swing Backwards.* Overbalance in the handstand, as explained in the last exercise, but retain the grasp and swing backwards. This movement may be done with ordinary, combined, or reverse grasp; with reverse or combined grasp it is easy, but a little dangerous at first, as the strain on the grasp is considerable, especially from a handstand with straight arms. With ordinary grasp the movement is difficult; you must let the weight drop down past the bar, and at the same time shift the grasp with a sudden movement of the wrists so that when the weight comes on the arms you have the hands in a proper position to support it. It is impossible to obtain more than a moderate swing by means of the overthrow with ordinary grasp; but I have seen a sufficient swing obtained in this way to enable the movement to be followed by a "back-up" (see § 305).

§ 251. *From the Handstand, High Front Vault Left.* From the handstand, overbalance, as described in § 249, then let go with the left hand, throw the left shoulder sharply forward, throw the head up and drop the legs past the bar just in front of it and alight as if you were finishing an ordinary front vault. The high front vault may be done from a handstand with bent arms or straight arms; it is a most important exercise to learn thoroughly, because it is the best way of saving yourself if you pitch suddenly in a handstand and find you are overbalanced, as will appear later.

§ 252. *From the Handstand, Squat to Ground.* From the handstand, overbalance in the same direction as for an overthrow, then press from the hands, let go, throw the head and shoulders sharply up and squat over the bar to the ground. This exercise is difficult and, at first, dangerous. As preliminary practice, you may do a handstand on the parallel bars at the further end (see Chapter IV.), placing a string across the bars in front of the hands, and try to squat over the string. When you can do this, you may try to squat over the horse without pommels from a handstand, you will not hurt your feet much if you do catch them on the horse, whereas on the bar it is very painful. When you can do the exercise on the horse, you are not likely to fail on the bar. I have seen a squat done from the handstand with a hollow back throughout the movement as in a sheep jump on the horse, but this is extremely difficult.

§ 253. *From the Handstand, Straddle to Ground.* This is just like the exercise described in the last paragraph, except that you straddle instead of squatting. Once you have learnt the squat from the handstand you will have little difficulty in learning the straddle. In both exercises you must endeavour to hollow the back completely before you alight.

KNEE AND SEAT CIRCLES, ETC.

§ 254. *From the Riding Seat, Right Leg Forward, Knee Circle Backwards.* From the riding seat mentioned, grasp the bar with both hands with ordinary grasp, throw the weight backwards, at the same time hooking the right knee round the bar, and throwing the left leg as far to the rear as you can, let the body drop behind the bar with the arms perfectly straight, continue the swing, and pass right round the bar, returning to the position from which you started. You will, of course, while you are underneath the bar, be in a leaning hang on the right knee. You may, for this exercise, grasp the bar with the hands one on each side of the right leg, or with both hands either to the left or right of the right leg, so that the exercise is possible in three positions. Similar movements may be done with combined or reverse grasp ; but they are somewhat constrained.

§ 255. *From the Riding Seat, Right Leg Forward, Knee Circle Forwards.* From the riding seat, grasp the bar with reverse grasp, throw the weight forwards, at the same time hooking the right knee round the bar, and throwing the left leg as far to the rear as you can, let the body drop in front of the bar with the arms perfectly straight, continue the swing, and pass right round the bar, returning to the position from which you started. You will, of course, while underneath the bar, be in a leaning hang on the right knee with

reverse grasp. Like the knee circle backwards, this exercise may be done in three positions, with the right leg
between the hands or outside the hands on either side.
Similar circles may be done with ordinary or combined
grasp; but they are rather constrained.

§ 256. *From the Side Seat, Seat Circle on Knees Backwards.* From the side seat, grasp the bar with both hands
in ordinary grasp, throw the weight backwards, hooking
both knees round the bar, let the body drop behind the bar
with the arms straight, continue the swing, and pass right
round the bar, returning to the position from which you
started; you pass, of course, through a leaning hang on
both knees. You may do this exercise with both legs
between the hands, with one leg between the hands and
one outside the hands, with both hands between the legs,
or with both hands on either side of the legs; in all, therefore, in six positions. Similar exercises may be done with
combined or reverse grasp; but they are rather constrained.

§ 257. *From the Side Seat, Seat Circle on Knees Forwards.* From the side seat, grasp the bar with both hands
in reverse grasp, throw the weight forward with straight
arms, at the same hooking both knees round the bar, let
the weight drop in front of the bar with straight arms, con-
tinne the swing, and pass right round the bar, returning to
the position whence you started. This exercise, like the
seat circle on the knees backwards, may be done in six
positions. Similar exercises may be done with ordinary or
combined grasp; but they are constrained and a little
dangerous at first.

§ 258. Almost all the exercises described in §§ 254–257
are easy. If after any of these circles you wish to come to
a rest, and remain there, you must straighten the leg, or
legs, hooked round the bar, just before you finish the circle,

and come to the proper position as you reach the rest. It is very difficult to regain the balance if you keep the leg, or legs, hooked round the bar too long.

§ 259. *From the Riding Seat, Mill Circle Backwards.* This exercise is just like a knee circle backwards, except that you do not hook one knee round the bar, but keep the legs straight, and keep the bar between the thighs close to the fork. Like a knee circle, it may be done with the hands in three positions. These exercises are easiest with the ordinary grasp, but may also be done with combined grasp. I doubt their being possible with reverse grasp.

§ 260. *From the Riding Seat, Mill Circle Forwards.* This exercise is like the knee circle forwards, but is done with straight knees, the bar being between the thighs. Like a knee circle forwards, it may be done with the hands in three positions. These exercises are easiest with reverse grasp, but may be done with combined or ordinary grasp.

§ 261. *Free Mill Circles.* Mill circles done without letting the legs touch the bar are called "free mill circles." Free mill circles backwards with ordinary grasp, or forwards with reverse grasp, are not difficult; but either way with combined grasp they are difficult, and I doubt its being possible to do a free mill circle backwards with reverse grasp, or forwards with ordinary grasp; and I doubt its being possible to do a free mill circle with the right leg over the bar to the left of the hands.

§ 262. *From the Side Seat, Free Seat Circle Backwards.* This exercise is like a seat circle backwards on the knees, except that you do not hook the knees round the bar, but keep the knees straight, and pass round the bar without touching it with the legs. It may be done with the legs between the hands, or the hands between the legs, or with one hand between the legs, and one outside, that is, in all, in four positions. I doubt its being possible, except with ordinary grasp. None of the free seat circles backwards are easy. If you wish to do a free seat circle backwards with the legs between the hands, start in the back rest, raise the feet to the half lever, and instantly throw the weight back boldly ; as soon as the weight begins to rise in front of the bar, hollow the back sharply, and at the same time shift the grasp of the hands, so that you bring the wrists above the bar with a sudden movement, and return to the back rest. The sharp hollowing of the back will release the strain on the hands for an instant, and it is at that instant that you must accomplish the shift of the grasp. The secret of the exercise lies entirely in hollowing the back, and shifting the grasp simultaneously, and in accomplishing these simultaneous movements at exactly the right time. A similar sharp hollowing of the back, and sudden shift of the grasp, is the secret of many other exercises on the bar. The movement of the hands in shifting the grasp is like the movement in feathering an oar. Beginners, not only in this exercise, but in all similar exercises, almost always hollow the back and shift the grasp too late. Free seat circles backwards in other positions are done in a similar manner, but the hollowing of the back is a little less vigorous. A seat circle backwards with the legs between the hands may be done with a hollow back throughout the movement, letting the seat remain in contact with the bar. This circle may be done with ordinary combined or reverse grasp ; it must be done very rapidly with a bold swing.

§ 263. *From the Side Seat, Free Seat Circle Forwards.* This exercise is like a seat circle forwards on the knees, except that you do not hook the knees round the bar, but keep the knees straight, and pass round the bar without touching it with the legs. Like the free seat circle backwards, it is possible in four positions. I doubt its being possible, except with the reverse grasp. The most important position is with the legs between the hands, so that you practically start from the back rest. To do this exercise you must raise the legs to the half lever momentarily, carrying them more to the front than is possible in a stationary position, then drop boldly, keeping the legs at right angles to the body all the time. If you wish to return to the back rest, it is not very difficult, and you do not want very much swing; if, however, you wish to clear the bar completely, and alight after the circle, or continue with another circle, you want a very good swing. The free seat circle forwards to ground, or followed by a second free seat circle forwards, are fine exercises; they require a fairly strong grasp. A free seat circle forwards with the legs between the hands may be done with a hollow back. You must begin almost as if to do the free seat circle described above; but, the moment the weight begins to drop, hollow the back sharply.

§ 264. I have described the exercises dealt with in §§ 254–263 as beginning from a seat in order to group them more easily; they may, of course, be begun from rests or free rests, and if you begin from a seat you come to a rest momentarily as you start the circle.

§ 265. The expressions "forward circle" and "backward circle" have been used several times in the last few paragraphs, and I may now explain the general meaning of these expressions. Whenever in an exercise the weight is carried round the bar, and at the same time the body makes a revolution about an axis of its own parallel to the bar (in other words, when you turn head over heels yourself), the movement is called a circle. If, while the weight is above the bar, it is moving from behind the bar towards the front of the bar, the circle is a "forward circle;" if in the opposite direction, a "backward circle." If Fig. 17 represents a cross section of the bar, the point B being in front of the bar, circles with the arrow are forward circles; circles in the other direction backward circles. The use of the word "circle" is a little loose in this respect, that it does not always indicate a complete revolution.

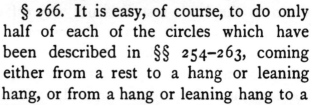

Fig. 17.

§ 266. It is easy, of course, to do only half of each of the circles which have been described in §§ 254–263, coming either from a rest to a hang or leaning hang, or from a hang or leaning hang to a rest. These exercises are discussed in the next few paragraphs.

§ 267. *From Leaning Hang on Right Knee, Half Knee Circle Forwards.* Come to the leaning hang mentioned, take a slight swing by swinging the left leg, and do a half knee circle forwards to a riding rest, or, if the leg is outside the hands, to a front rest with the right leg over the bar. This is the very easiest way of reaching a rest on a high bar. The exercise may be done with ordinary, reverse, or combined grasp.

§ 268. *From the Leaning Hang on Both Knees, Half Seat Circle Forwards on Knees.* Come to the leaning hang mentioned, take a slight swing, and do a half seat circle forwards on the knees coming to a rest. This exercise is easy, except when both legs are on the same side of the hands. It may be done with ordinary, reverse, or combined grasp.

§ 269. *From the Hang with Legs Astride Bar, Half Mill Circle Forwards.* Come to the hang mentioned with the legs straight, and the feet very little above the bar, take a slight swing, and do a half mill circle forwards to a riding rest, or, if the leg behind the bar is not between the hands, to a front rest with one leg over the bar. This exercise may be done with ordinary, reverse, or combined grasp ; it differs slightly from the last half of a mill circle, because in a mill circle you keep the bar close to the fork all the time, whereas in the half mill circle from the hang your feet are close to the bar at the beginning of the movement.

§ 270. *From the Back Hang, Heels to Bar, Half Free Seat Circle Forwards to Back Rest.* From the back hang mentioned, which is more fully described in § 207, take a slight swing, and do a half free seat circle forwards to the back rest ; the exercise may be done with ordinary, combined, or reverse grasp. The movement is rather different from the last half of a free seat circle, because in the complete circle you keep the bar close to the seat all the time, whereas in the half circle from the hang your feet are close to the bar at the beginning of the movement. You may come to the free back rest with this movement, and press strongly from the hands, and alight.

§ 271. Half free seat circles forwards, similar to that described in the last paragraph, may be done from a hang with the legs astride one arm or with the legs astride both arms.

§ 272. The easiest way of learning all the exercises described in §§ 267–271 with the ordinary grasp is to begin from the rest which you intend to reach, do a half circle backwards, and then the half circle forwards on the return swing. In doing the half circle backwards preparatory to the exercises described in §§ 269–271 you must, of course, let the waist bend well, so that the feet come almost level with the bar. Half circles backwards from rests done in this manner are of considerable importance, as will appear later.

§ 273. *From the Leaning Hang on Right Knee, Half Knee Circle Backwards.* Come to the leaning hang mentioned, take a slight swing by swinging the left leg, and do a half knee circle backwards, bringing you to a riding rest, or, if the right leg is outside the hands, to a front rest with the right leg over the bar. This exercise may be done with ordinary, combined, or reverse grasp.

§ 274. *From the Leaning Hang on Both Knees, Half Seat Circle on Knees Backwards.* Come to the leaning hang mentioned, take a slight swing, and do a half seat circle backwards, coming to a side seat on the bar. This exercise may be done with ordinary, combined, or reverse grasp.

§ 275. *From the Hang with Legs Astride Bar, Half Mill Circle Backwards.* Come to the hang mentioned with the legs straight and the feet very little above the bar, take a slight swing, and do a half mill circle backwards, coming to a riding rest, or, if the leg behind the bar is outside the hands, to a front rest with one leg over the bar. This exercise may be done with ordinary, combined, or reverse grasp. You must hollow the back rather sharply as you begin the movement.

§ 276. *From the Back Hang, Heels to Bar, Half Free Seat Circle Backwards.* From the hang mentioned, take a slight swing and do a half free seat circle backwards to the back rest. You must hollow the back and shift the grasp very sharply in doing this movement. At first you will only be able to come to the back rest with bent arms. The exercise may be done with ordinary, combined, or reverse grasp.

§ 277. Exercises similar to that described in the last paragraph may be done from a hang with legs astride one arm or astride both arms.

SWINGING.

§ 278. *Forward and Backward Swings.* A swing in which the weight passes from behind the bar to the front of the bar is called a forward swing, and a swing in the other direction is called a backward swing. It may be pointed out that, in a backward circle, you swing forwards while underneath the bar, and that, in a forward circle, you swing backwards while underneath the bar.

§ 279. *From the Rest, Long Underswing.* From the rest, throw the body and legs to the rear, let the body and legs sink behind the bar till you hang with straight arms, and then swing forward. This movement is, of course, very easy with the ordinary or combined grasp. You must, however, be careful at first that you do not take too much swing. With the reverse grasp this movement is very difficult, and requires great strength of grasp.

§ 280. You may do a long underswing on a low bar, but the movement is somewhat different from that done in the long underswing on a high bar. It is easiest from a standing position. You must stand well behind the bar, grasping it at arm's length, with the shoulders rather lower than the bar and the back hollow, so that the feet are behind the shoulders. Then spring from the feet, bend at the waist and swing forward, keeping the legs straight and the feet throughout the movement a few inches from the ground, so that, until the feet pass under the bar, you bend gradually a little more and more at the waist, and then gradually unbend, so that at the extremity of the swing the back is nearly hollow. A long underswing may also be done on the low bar from the rest, bending at waist as the body drops below the bar. A long underswing on the low bar from the stand is not difficult with reverse grasp.

§ 281. *From the Rest, Drop Back.* From the rest, throw the feet slightly to the rear, then let the body sink behind the bar, keeping the arms perfectly straight, at the same time bend at the waist and raise the feet to the bar, so that you come to a hang with the feet to the bar. The feet throughout the movement never drop lower than their original position. When the feet reach the bar, if you have done the movement properly, you will still be swinging forward, and you will find that the feet have an irresistible tendency to swing away from the bar, and at first you will be unable to stop them, so that they will swing right away, and you will come to a hang at full length. After some practice, however, you will find that, after the feet have gone some inches from the bar, you will be able to stop them, and, just as you begin to swing back again, to bring the feet close to the bar once more. The drop back from the rest may be done with ordinary combined or reverse grasp; with the reverse grasp it is difficult, but not nearly so difficult as the long underswing. A drop back from the rest may be followed by a great variety of movements, as will appear later. Some of these movements are dealt with in the next few paragraphs.

§ 282. On a low bar you may do a movement similar to the drop back from the rest, starting from a standing position. Stand behind the bar, holding the bar at arm's length, and with the body upright, or, if anything, leaning slightly back, spring from the feet almost to a free rest, but not quite, and then swing forward, raising the feet in front of the bar at once. This movement is called a " drop swing."

§ 283. *From the Rest, Drop Back and Short Underswing to Ground.* Begin as in the exercise described in § 281, then, the moment the feet begin to leave the bar, bend the arms, hollow the back sharply, and let go. You will then fly through the air and alight some distance in front of the bar. You should practise the short underswing to the ground, placing a string in front of the bar and parallel to it and endeavouring to clear this string. You may begin with the string quite low, but with practice you should clear a string quite as high as, or higher than, the bar. If you can clear a string level with the bar and about 3 feet from it and alight steadily, you may consider, if your style is otherwise good, that you have done a good short underswing to the ground. The short underswing to the ground is a most important exercise to practise, as it forms perhaps the most usual way of leaving the bar, and is also an excellent introductory exercise to the "upstart" and "back-up," which are two of the principal exercises on the bar.

§ 284. *From the Riding Seat, Right Leg Forward, Drop Back, and Short Underswing to Ground.* Do a half mill circle backwards, as explained in § 272, bringing the feet to the bar in the course of the movement, but just before you are exactly underneath the bar bring the right leg from behind the bar to join the left; you will then be exactly in the same position as if you had done a drop back from the rest, and you come to the ground as described in the last paragraph. If you begin with the hands one on each side of the right leg, you must, of course, bring the right leg through between the arms; some men can bring the leg through without bending the knee, and, of course, if you can manage it, that is the right way to do the exercise. If you begin with the hands on one side of the right leg, you must keep it as close to the hands as you can while bringing it in front of the bar; every one can learn to keep the leg straight throughout this movement.

§ 285. *From the Side Seat, Drop Back, and Short Underswing to Ground.* This exercise is just like that

described in the last paragraph, except that you begin with
a half free seat circle backwards, and then bring both feet
from behind the bar.   If you start with the legs between
the hands it is very difficult to avoid bending the knees,
but some men can accomplish it.   If you start with the
hands between the legs you can easily keep them straight,
because there is no objection to straddling them as wide as
you find necessary to avoid bending.

§ 286. The expression "drop back" is used in several
senses; it is used to describe the movement explained in
§ 281, and also to mean a half mill circle or seat circle
backwards.   Where such a half circle is followed by some
movement, which must be begun from a hang with both
feet in front of the bar, it is unnecessary to mention that
the feet are to be brought from behind the bar, as that is
implied.   The various meanings of the expression will not
be found to lead to any confusion.

§ 287. *Swings from the Hang, or from the Ground.*   It is
most important to learn to take a good swing on the bar
either from a hang, or direct from the ground with a jump,
but it is extremely difficult to describe the exact movement
by which the swing should be taken.   I shall, in this
paragraph, describe one method of taking a swing, and
then, in subsequent paragraphs, endeavour to explain how
this may be varied according to the position you are in
when you want to begin your swing.   Stand facing the bar
about eighteen inches or two feet from it, jump to a hang
with ordinary grasp with the arms slightly bent, so that the
upper arms are about at right angles to the forearms; you
will then find that you have a slight swing.   Remain in this
position until you have reached the extremity of your
forward swing, then, as you swing back again, let the arms
straighten gradually, so that when you reach the extremity

of your backward swing the arms are almost, but not quite, straight; then, as you swing forward again, bend the arms sharply, raise the body and legs in front of the bar almost in the same way as if you intended to carry the body over the bar, and when you have nearly reached the extremity of the forward swing hollow the back sharply, and, with a vigorous movement, throw the body and legs to the front and straighten the arms, retain the grasp and swing backwards. The latter part of this movement is very like the short underswing to the ground, except that you do not let go. It seems rather unnecessary to bend the arms in the manner described and then straighten them again pre- paratory to the final bending of the arms, and I have never been able to see exactly why it helps you in taking your swing; it certainly does, however. Probably it gets the muscles of the shoulders into a better position for the final effort.

§ 288. You may take a swing with the reverse grasp in the same way as with an ordinary grasp, but, as you throw the feet and body forward, you must shift the grasp, raising the wrists in front of the bar. It is at first much more difficult to get a good swing with the reverse grasp than with the ordinary grasp, but, after a time, you will find that it is really easier, for the following reason. If, with the ordinary grasp, when you throw the body and legs up in front of the bar, you raise the weight much above the bar, you will be unable to retain the grasp in the return swing without bending your arms, so that the swing you can obtain is limited in this way. On the other hand, there is no such limit with the reverse grasp, because, after shifting the grasp in the manner described above, the hands are in the best position for retaining the grasp on the return swing. You may, therefore, in taking the swing with reverse grasp, make the movement, throwing the body and legs up in front of the bar, rather later than in taking a swing with the ordinary grasp, and throw the body much higher. In this way it is possible to throw the body so high that you reach a momentary handstand, and then you can return as if you were doing a long circle forwards, in which case, of course, you have the best swing it is possible to get. This movement is further discussed in § 301. It is, of course, possible to do a similar movement with the ordinary grasp if you shift the grasp, reaching the handstand with the ordinary grasp, but then you will be unable to return, at any rate, with more than a very moderate swing. You may take a swing with a combined grasp in a similar way, shifting the grasp, of course, with the hand which has the reverse grasp. You can get a better swing with the combined grasp than with the ordinary grasp, but not such a good swing as you can with a reverse grasp.

§ 289. You may take a swing with ordinary, combined, or reverse grasp, beginning from a hang with the arms straight and the body perfectly still. The movement is very like that hitherto described. You bend the arms and raise the body and legs, hollow the back, and throw the body and legs to the front, and high. It is, however, much more difficult to get a good swing in this manner than with a slight preliminary swing.

§ 290. You may also take a swing with ordinary, combined, or reverse grasp with a jump from the ground, starting about eighteen inches or two feet behind the bar, and omitting the preliminary swing forwards and backwards, described in § 287; you jump up, bend the arms, and raise the body and legs in the first swing forwards. With the ordinary grasp it is perhaps rather easier to get a good swing in this way than after a preliminary swing, but with combined or reverse grasp it is much more difficult.

§ 291. *From the Rest, Drop Back and Swing Back with Short Underswing.* From the rest, drop back, and when the feet leave the bar, bend the arms and hollow the back sharply, in the manner described in § 287, throwing the body and legs to the front; straighten the arms and swing back. The movement is almost exactly similar to the drop back and short underswing to the ground, except that you retain the grasp.

§ 292. *From the Side Seat, or Side Riding Seat, Drop Back, and Swing Back with Short Underswing.* Begin from the seat, as if you intended to drop back and do a short underswing to the ground, as described in §§ 284, 285, but, instead of finishing the movement, continue as described in the last paragraph.

§ 293. *From the Rest, Roll Forward and Swing Back.* This movement is like the roll forward, explained in § 232, done quickly, so that, when the thighs leave the bar, you swing backwards.

UPSTARTS.

§ 294. *Hang, Swing, Upstart.* Hang, and take a swing; as you swing forward, and a little after you have passed the vertical position below the bar, raise the feet to the bar, keeping the legs and arms straight, so that the feet come to the bar just before you reach the extremity of the forward swing. Then, as you begin to swing back, press strongly with the arms and, without bending them, raise the body behind the bar, at the same time dropping the feet, so that you come to the rest. Success in this exercise depends entirely on making the effort to rise at exactly the right time. Beginners generally make the effort much too soon.

After you straighten the arms in taking the swing you will, of course, swing backwards; during this swing you must keep the arms perfectly straight and the body in a straight line with arms, and the head exactly between the arms. As you swing back, therefore, you should keep the eyes on the ground. Beginners generally look at the bar when they reach the extremity of the backward swing, but this brings the body out of line with the arms, and checks the swing. After you have straightened the arms in taking the swing you have absolutely nothing to do till you pass the vertical position in the next forward swing except to hold the bar and keep the muscles of the legs braced so that they do not bend, otherwise you should simply hang like a log. You do not require a very big swing.

The upstart may be done with ordinary, combined, or reverse grasp; it is much easiest with the ordinary grasp. In doing an upstart with the reverse grasp it is particularly important to keep the eyes on the ground during the backward swing; you must also be particularly careful not to bend the arms at all. Beginners are very apt to bend the arms, owing to a feeling of insecurity in the grasp during the forward swing, but, after a time, you will find that, although you will at the extremity of the forward swing hang almost by the tips of the fingers, your grasp is really quite safe.

§ 295. *From the Rest, Short Upstart.* From the rest, do a drop back; the feet will, as explained in § 281, pass away from the bar, let them swing well away and rise considerably higher than the bar, then bring them back, and, the moment the feet return to the bar, press from the hands and return to the rest, as in the upstart described in the last paragraph. It is perhaps a little more difficult to do an upstart in this manner than with a swing as described in the last paragraph;

but, if you have no one to show you how to do an upstart, I should advise you to begin with this one, because there is less difficulty in knowing when to make your effort. The short upstart may of course be done with ordinary, reverse, or combined grasp.

§ 296. *From the Rest, Long Upstart.* From the rest, do a long underswing, and then an upstart as described in § 294. A long upstart may, of course, be done on a low bar, starting either from a stand or from a rest, as described in § 280.

§ 297. *From the Side Seat or Riding Seat, Drop Back and Upstart.* From the position mentioned, drop back and bring the feet in front of the bar as if preparatory to a short underswing to ground, as explained in §§ 284, 285, but, instead of doing a short underswing to ground, do an upstart. These movements are of considerable variety, because in starting from the side seat you may place the hands altogether in six positions, or from the riding seat in three ; as you may in a seat or knee circle backwards, as explained in §§ 254, 256.

§ 298. It must be observed that the word "upstart" is used a little vaguely ; it generally means the last part of the movement alone, from the moment when the feet are brought to the bar ; but the phrases "short upstart" and "long upstart" are used to mean drop back and upstart, and long underswing and upstart, respectively.

SWING AND KNEE, OR SEAT CIRCLES, ETC.

§ 299. The half knee, mill, or seat circles forwards, explained in §§ 267–271, may be combined with a swing. You swing, and raise the feet to the bar, as if to do an upstart, and then, at the same moment as that at which, in an upstart, you would make your effort to rise behind the bar, pass one leg, or both legs, behind the bar, as the case may be, and do the corresponding half circle, rising to a rest or seat on the bar.　For example—

(i.) Hang, Swing, Pass Right Leg between Hands and Half Knee Circle Forwards to Riding Rest.　This is an easy combination; similar combinations can be done with the right leg on either side of the hands.

(ii.) Hang, Swing, Pass Right Leg between Hands, and Half Free Mill Circle Forwards to Riding Rest.　This is a little more difficult than the last exercise; as in the upstart, the timing of the movements is the secret of success.　A similar movement may be done with the right leg outside the arms on the right; it is difficult to do this without letting the leg touch the bar.

(iii.) Hang, Swing, Pass Both Legs between Hands and Half Seat Circle on Knees or Half Free Seat Circle Forwards to Back Rest.　This exercise with the half free seat circle is very effective; you want a good deal of swing, if you do it well, you may come clear over the bar to a momentary back rest with the legs in half lever, and then push strongly from the hands and alight.

(iv.) Hang, Swing, Pass Both Legs behind Bar outside Hands, and Half Seat Circle Forwards on Knees, or Half Free Seat Circle Forwards with Hands between Legs.　This exercise with the half free seat circle forwards is very effective; the whole movement should, of course, be done with straight legs.　If you intend to remain in the side seat, you must let go with the hands rather before you come completely to the seat, and place the hands outside the legs.

All the exercises described in this paragraph may be done with ordinary, reverse, or combined grasp.　They may also be done after a drop back from the rest; also after doing a drop back from the side seat or riding seat, and bringing the feet in front of the bar, as described in §§ 284–286.

CLEAR CIRCLE, SHORT CIRCLE, FRONT CIRCLE AND HAND CIRCLE.

§ 300. *From the Hang, with a Slight Swing, Clear Circle.* Hang with a slight swing, and go through the same preliminary movements that you would in preparing to take a swing, as described in § 287. That is, have the arms bent at the forward end of your slight swing, let them straighten gradually as you swing back, then, as you swing forward, bend them again sharply and raise the body and legs in front of the bar ; but this last movement you must do a little sooner than you would if you were going to take a swing. Then continue your movement, letting the body and legs pass over the bar in the same direction as in the slow circle, described in § 231. At the same time hollow the back sharply, shift the grasp in a manner similar to that described in § 262, and come to the free rest. The exercise may be done with ordinary, combined, or reverse grasp. At first you will find that you will be able just to get over the bar without touching it, but that you will not get the body high enough nor the grasp sufficiently shifted to reach the free rest, and you will simply drop again to a hang.

§ 301. The method described in the last paragraph is the easiest method of doing a clear circle with the combined or reverse grasp, but with the ordinary grasp it is rather easier to do the exercise from a jump, omitting the first swing forwards and backwards, and proceeding as if you were going to take a swing in the manner described in § 290, bending the arms, however, a trifle later, and throwing the body and legs up higher and a little sooner. The clear circle may also be done with ordinary, combined, or reverse grasp, from a perfectly still hang. Again, with ordinary, combined, or reverse grasp, beginning either with a slight swing or with a jump, you may do a clear circle to a handstand with either bent or straight arms, as has already been indicated in § 288. These movements, I need scarcely say, are of extreme difficulty.

§ 302. *From the Rest, Short Circle.* From the rest, throw the legs back to a free rest with the legs some little way from the bar, then drop back in somewhat the same manner as if you were going to do a short underswing, but do not bend nearly so much at the waist, so that in the hang the thighs are opposite the bar ; then continue your swing and let the body and legs pass round and over the bar, at the same time sharply hollowing the back and shifting the grasp, returning to the free rest again. This exercise is of great importance, and is by no means easy. It is possible, by taking plenty of swing and hollowing the back very early in the movement and very sharply, to come to the handstand at the end of the movement instead of to the free rest, though this is of course very difficult. The short circle may be done with ordinary, combined, or reverse grasp. With the reverse grasp, however, it is very difficult, and, at the best, a constrained movement, as it is impossible to retain the grasp of the bar if you take at all much swing.

§ 303. *From the Rest, Front Circle.* From the rest, let the body drop in front of the bar, at the same time letting the body bend at the waist, and the thighs remain in contact with the bar, so that you come to a leaning hang on the front of both thighs ; continue the movement, and rise again behind the bar to the rest. As you pass under the bar the thighs will leave the bar, and, as you rise, your stomach will come in contact with it, so that you are in the position described in § 243, as preparatory to vaults from the rest, and, from that position, you may rise again to the rest. The front circle may be done with ordinary, reverse, or combined grasp ; it is easiest with the ordinary grasp. In doing the exercise with the ordinary grasp, you must shift the hands as you begin the movement, passing the wrists under the bar, so that you have the hands in a proper position for reaching the rest.

§ 304. *From the Back Rest, Hand Circle.* From the back rest with reverse grasp, raise the legs and drop to the bent arm rest, in that position swing back and pass round the bar, keeping the back hollow, and the bar in contact with the small of the back ; as you rise above the bar again, straighten the arms and return to the back rest. This is an easy movement ; in order to recover the back rest, you will have to bend a little at the waist as you rise above the bar. A hand circle may also be done with combined grasp.

THE BACK-UP.

§ 305. *Hang, and Back-Up.* Hang, and take as good a swing as you can, as explained in § 287. As you approach the end of your backward swing, press strongly from the hands and come to the rest. After the back is hollowed in taking the swing, it should be kept perfectly hollow throughout the whole movement. Success in the exercise depends almost entirely upon getting sufficient swing. At first, you will find that you will not be able to come to the rest, but that you will be able nearly to reach a free rest, with, however, the weight too low, and the legs too far forward. In fact, you will come to a position like this ⟍, whereas the free rest is like this ⟋. Accordingly, at first, you should follow the back-up with ordinary grasp by a short circle at once, or else you will come against the bar with a violent blow on the pit of the stomach. The back-up may be done with ordinary, combined, or reverse grasp ; it is easiest to accomplish with the ordinary grasp, but easiest to do well with the reverse grasp. In doing a back-up with the reverse grasp you should begin by throwing the feet and body almost to a handstand, as explained in §§ 288, 301, and then you will have such a swing that you will do the back-up almost without any further effort.

§ 306. *From the Rest, Drop Back and Back-Up with Short Underswing.* From the rest, drop back and swing back with a short underswing, as explained in § 291, and then rise to the rest as explained in the last paragraph. This exercise may be done with ordinary, combined, or reverse grasp, but with the reverse grasp it is exceedingly difficult.

§ 307. *From the Rest, Long Underswing and Back-Up.* From the rest, do a long underswing, and, keeping the back hollow, swing back and rise to the rest as explained in § 305. This is, at best, a somewhat cramped movement, as it is impossible to get sufficient swing in this way to do a back-up in good style; it can be done with ordinary, combined, or reverse grasp, but with the reverse grasp it is exceedingly difficult.

§ 308. *From the Seat or Riding Seat, Drop Back and Back-Up with Short Underswing.* You begin as explained in § 292, and then swing back and rise to the rest, as explained in § 306. This may be done with ordinary or combined grasp, but I do not think it is possible with reverse grasp.

§ 309. The expression "back-up" is sometimes used to indicate the complete movement, including the taking of the swing, sometimes the latter part of the movement alone.

LONG CIRCLES AND HALF LONG CIRCLES.

§ 310. *From the Handstand, Long Circle Backwards.* From the handstand, let the weight pass behind the bar, swing down in a long underswing, keeping the arms straight and the body and arms in a straight line, continue the swing, and, as you rise in front of the bar, hollow the back slightly, and, at the same time, shift the grasp and return to the hand-stand again. I have never seen a long circle backwards done with any but the ordinary grasp; it might, perhaps, be done with combined grasp; with reverse grasp it is quite impossible. It is not advisable to begin to learn the long circle by reaching a handstand and starting from that position; if you do, you run great risk; in the first place, the strain on the grasp, while passing under the bar, is consider-able, and you may slip off the bar altogether, in which case you will come to terrible grief; secondly, you may reach the handstand again, and then overbalance forwards; ir this happens, you ought at once to do a high front vault; but the chances are you will not have presence of mind to do this, and you will pitch on the top of your head; thirdly, you may fail to shift the grasp, and, after nearly reaching a handstand, fall in a heap on the top of the bar and break your jaw or a rib or two. Before attempting a long circle backwards, I should advise you, first, to learn the high front vault thoroughly on a low bar; secondly, to learn to do short circles to a handstand, not necessarily so as to be certain of reaching a handstand, but till you have learnt to do a high front vault without hesitation if you find yourself in a handstand overbalanced forwards. This, of course, you may learn on a low bar, so that you can get a friend to stand and save you from a fall. When you have confidence in this movement, try on a high bar to take as good a swing as you can, and then, as you swing forward, circle the bar to the free rest; as you raise the body in front of the bar, you must hollow the back sharply and shift the grasp sharply. At first, you will land with rather a crash on the bar, but that will be for want of shifting the hands properly. Then try and do the same movement to a handstand, by hollowing the back and shifting the grasp still sooner and more sharply. Be content to come to a handstand with bent arms until you are confident of doing the high front vault if you over-balance. Then, having reached the handstand with bent arms, throw the weight behind the bar, do a long under-swing, and return to the handstand with bent arms just as you have done from a swing, and you have done a long circle of a kind; you have now only gradually to increase the swing till at last you do your handstand with straight arms. I should, perhaps, say that it is hardly fair to ask any one to try and save you in a long circle. The only fall he can save is the fall forwards after overbalancing in the hand-stand, and it is almost impossible to save a big man from this fall, especially if he comes to the handstand with straight arms. The long circle backwards requires considerably less strength and dexterity than some of the exercises which I suggested ought to be learnt first, and many men, who are by no means good gymnasts, can do it, but they run con-siderable risk, and are, in my opinion, rather to be con-demned for their folly than admired for their daring.

§ 311. *From the Handstand with Reverse Grasp, Long Circle Forwards.* From the handstand, do an overthrow, retaining the grasp, and, as you swing back, do a back-up, and come again to the handstand. In this exercise the only danger is of not being able to hold on; the strain on the grasp, especially on a thick bar, is very great. I should recommend you not to try it till you can do a back-up with the reverse grasp, followed by a handstand, keeping the back hollow all the time. As soon as you can do this, the long circle forwards is practically learnt.

§ 312. *Half Long Circles.* This expression, "half long circle," means that you circle the bar as in a long circle, passing under the bar with a swing at arm's length; but either not starting from a handstand, or not reaching a handstand, or neither starting from a handstand, nor coming to a handstand. Thus the exercise, explained in § 310 as preparatory to a long circle backwards, in which you take a swing, and then circle the bar to a free rest, would be described as "swing and half long circle backwards to free rest," and the next exercise, described in that paragraph, would be described as "swing and half long circle backwards to handstand." Again, you may begin from the handstand as if to do a long circle backwards, but, instead of returning to the handstand, check the swing a little, and shift the grasp rather late, coming to a free rest; this movement is described as "from the handstand, half long circle backwards to free rest." .From a swing, a half long circle backwards may be done with reverse or combined grasp to the free rest or even to a handstand with bent arms. From the handstand with bent arms with reverse grasp, it is possible to do a long underswing, and I have seen this combined with a half long circle backwards to the handstand with bent arms so as to constitute a sort of bastard long circle backwards with reverse grasp. This exercise is, however, of the most extreme difficulty, and requires extraordinary strength of grasp; it is, of course, at the best, a somewhat constrained movement.

COMBINATION OF EXERCISES.

§ 313. Leg circles, and squatting and straddling movements, may be combined with knee, mill, and seat circles, and half circles, and it is not difficult to devise such combinations. In doing these combinations, whenever a leg circle is followed by, or follows, a knee, seat, or mill circle, you should begin the second movement just before the first is finished, and in that way you often avoid having to recover your balance in the rest, which is the great difficulty about all these movements; however, the less you do this, provided you do not check the even flow of your movement, the better in point of style your exercise will be. It should be clear that you could stop in the rest if you wished. The following examples will serve to explain how these combinations may be done, and how the balance should be managed.

(i.) From the Rest, Half Right Circle with Right Leg (bringing you to a free riding rest; when you are in this position you should be just enough overbalanced backwards to prevent there being any effort to avoid falling forwards). Mill Circle Backwards, Half Mill Circle Backwards, Half Mill Circle Forwards (see § 272), Half Right Circle with Left Leg (you should begin the half right circle with the left leg just before you come to the riding rest, and when you reach the back rest you should again be just off the balance backwards). Free Seat Circle Backwards, Half Free Seat Circle Backwards, Half Free Seat Circle Forwards to Ground (see § 270).

(ii.) From the Rest with Reverse Grasp, Squat to Momentary Back Rest with Legs in Half Lever, and Free Seat Circle Forwards to Ground (see § 263). This is a difficult combination.

(iii.) From the Rest, Half Right Circle with Both Legs (bringing you to the back rest; you should now be just overbalanced backwards), Free Seat Circle Backwards, and Half Left Circle with Both Legs to Ground with a Quarter Left Turn. The last part of this exercise is difficult; the legs should not touch the bar after the free seat circle is begun; the last part of the movement is like a rear vault backwards on the horse (see § 55).

§ 314. Half knee, mill, or seat circles backwards may be

followed by an upstart or back-up, as has been explained in §§ 297, 308, or, after bringing the leg, or legs, from behind the bar, and then passing one leg, or both legs, behind the bar again, by half knee, mill, or seat circles forwards, as has been explained in § 299. Again, after a forward swing, you may pass one leg, or both legs, behind the bar, and then do a half knee, mill, or seat circle forwards, as has been explained in § 299. Again, after a forward swing, or drop back, you may pass one leg, or both legs, behind the bar, and then, as you swing forwards again, do a half knee, mill, or seat circle backwards (see §§ 273–277) ; these movements are not very effective, but they are excellent practice for the movements described in the next two paragraphs.

§ 315. You may jump to a hang on the bar from some little distance behind it, and instantly pass one leg, or both legs, behind the bar, and do a half knee, mill, or seat circle backwards. You must get the leg, or legs, behind the bar before you pass under the bar in the forward swing which you obtain by jumping to the hang. You may, of course, pass the leg, or legs, behind the bar between the hands or outside them. Similar exercises may be done from the hang with a slight swing.

§ 316. You may drop back from the rest, and, a little before you are exactly underneath the bar, pass one leg, or both legs, behind the bar, and then, continuing the movement, do a half knee, mill, or seat circle backwards. These movements, which are very pretty, are very similar to those described in the last paragraph.

§ 317. You may, from a riding seat or side seat, do a half free mill or seat circle forwards, and just before you pass under the bar bring the one leg or both legs in front of the bar, and, continuing the movement, do an upstart. These exercises are difficult, but very pretty.

§ 318. A clear circle or short circle may be followed by a short circle, or by a drop back, or long underswing; you must endeavour to show the free rest distinctly between the movements with the arms perfectly straight, and the back hollow, and with the body well clear of the bar, and the feet high; indeed, the position should be very like a free front lever on the horse.

§ 319. A front circle may be followed by a vault, leg circle, squatting or straddling movement, drop back, long underswing, short circle, or handstand. If you intend to follow a front circle by a drop back or short circle you should show the free rest distinctly between the movements with the arms straight, and the back hollow, and with the body well clear of the bar, and the feet high, though not quite so high as after a short circle. Vaults, and squat or straddle to the ground, are easy after a front circle, and at the same time effective. Leg circles, and squatting or straddling movements to a rest, on the other hand, are rather difficult, the tendency being to get the weight too high.

§ 320. The upstart may be followed by vaults, leg circles, squatting and straddling movements, drop back, long underswing, short circle, front circle, or handstand. At first you may do these movements letting the stomach or thighs come in contact with the bar for an instant as you finish the upstart, and thus getting a fresh impetus; but all these exercises can and should be done without this. If you intend to follow the upstart by a drop back, or short circle, or squat or straddle to the ground, you should be careful to show the free rest between the movements distinctly with the arms perfectly straight, the back hollow, the body well clear of the bar, and the feet fairly high, though not so high as after a short circle.

§ 321. The following are examples; of the combinations discussed in §§ 313–320—

(i.) Hang, Swing, Upstart, Short Circle, Short Upstart, Front Circle, Long Upstart, Half Right Circle with Both Legs, Clear Seat Circle Backwards to Back Rest, Pause, Squat Back with Both Legs (to free rest), Short Upstart, and Straddle to Ground.

(ii.) Hang with Reverse Grasp, Swing, Upstart, Squat Forwards with Right Leg, Free Mill Circle Forwards, Half Right Circle with Left Leg (this half circle should be done before the mill circle is fairly finished, so that you come to the back rest without pausing at all in the riding rest), Pause, and take Ordinary Grasp, Half Right Circle with Both Legs to Free Rest, Short Upstart, Long Upstart, and Front Vault Right.

(iii.) Hang, Swing, Bring Right Leg Behind B ir outside Right Hand, Half Free Mill Circle Forwards to Rest with Right Leg Over Bar, Half Right Circle with Right Leg, Half Right Circle with Both Legs, Drop Back, Upstart, Straddle to Straddle Rest, Free Seat Circle Backwards, Drop Back, Upstart, Front Circle, and Squat to Ground. After the half mill circle forwards in this exercise, you will find yourself much in the same position as if you were doing a right feint.

(iv.) Hang, Swing, Upstart, Handstand, and High Front Vault. If this exercise is properly done, the arms should be straight throughout the movement, and the back hollow after the free rest is reached. It is exceedingly difficult, however.

(v.) Jump to Bar, pass Both Legs behind Bar astride Arms, Half Free Seat Circle Backwards, Drop Back, Upstart, Drop Back, bringing Legs between Arms, and Half Seat Circle Backwards to Side Seat, Pause, and take Reverse Grasp, Half Free Seat Circle Forwards, bringing Legs between Arms, and Upstart, Front Circle, and Flank Vault Left to Ground.

§ 322. The back-up may be followed by all the movements by which an upstart may be followed, but, except the drop back and short circle, all such movements are very much more difficult after the back-up than after the upstart. Back-up, and vault, squat, or straddle to ground, are extremely difficult exercises with the ordinary grasp, and are very rarely accomplished; with the reverse grasp, they are, though far from easy, of considerably less difficulty. I have seen a back-up with the ordinary grasp followed by a handstand done with straight arms and a hollow back throughout the movement; but the man whom I saw do it was able to bend his back much more than most men, and that made it easier, of course. The back-up and handstand with reverse grasp is not so very difficult. If you can get to the handstand in front of the bar in taking the swing, or anywhere near it, there is no further difficulty, you practically do a long circle forwards. If you intend to follow a back-up by a short circle or drop back, you must endeavour to do your free rest between the movements with the arms straight, the back hollow, and the body well clear of the bar, and with the feet as high as possible. The following exercises introduce combinations with the back-up—

(i.) Jump to Bar, Back-Up, Short Circle, Drop Back, Back-Up, Short Upstart, Front Circle, Long Underswing, Bring the Right Leg Behind Bar to Left of Left Hand, Half Knee Circle Forwards, and Half Right Circle with Left Leg to Ground.

(ii.) Hang, Back-Up, Half Right Circle with Left Leg, Free Mill Circle Backwards, Drop Back, Back-Up, Short Circle, Drop Back, and Short Underswing to Ground.

(iii.) Hang with Reverse Grasp, Back-Up, Front Circle,

Overthrow, Back-Up, and Front Vault to Ground. The last part of this exercise is very nearly a long circle; you should hardly try it unless you can do a back-up and vault with reverse grasp from the hang.

§ 323. You may, as has been explained in §§ 301, 302, do a clear circle or short circle to a handstand; from the handstand, you may do a high front vault, overthrow, or squat, or straddle to the ground. These movements are, of course, extremely difficult, but they are very effective. You may also follow a short circle by a half leg circle, or squatting, or straddling movement. These combinations are very difficult, but exceedingly pretty; you must do your short circle very perfectly, so that you reach a free rest with the arms perfectly straight, the body almost horizontal, and the weight exactly over the bar, and then, without the slightest hesitation, do a half circle with one leg, or both legs, or squat to the back rest, or straddle to the straddle rest. After reaching the back rest, or riding or straddle rest, you are almost certain to overbalance backwards, so that practically you must follow these movements by a mill, or seat circle, or half circle, backwards.

§ 324. Long circles and half long circles may easily be brought into combination with the upstart, back-up, etc.; any movement which brings you to a handstand may, of course, be followed by a long circle backwards or forwards, according to your grasp. A long circle backwards may also be followed by an overthrow, or squat or straddle from the handstand, and it is not necessary, prior to such movements, to come to a stationary handstand.

CHANGING GRASP.

§ 325. The grasp can be changed from ordinary grasp to reverse grasp, or *vice versâ*, without turning, in various ways—

(i.) When you are in a side seat or side riding seat momentarily, it is, of course, easy to change the grasp with one hand or with both hands.

(ii.) The grasp may also be easily changed while doing leg circles, the hand raised to allow the leg or legs to pass, being put down with the other grasp.

(iii.) The grasp may be changed with either hand or both hands while in a free rest; for example: after an upstart with reverse grasp you may change to the ordinary grasp, and continue without pause, and you may do a similar change after a front circle or a back-up.

(iv.) The grasp may be changed while swinging; for example: hang with reverse grasp, and take a swing, and, when at the back end of the swing, change the grasp to ordinary grasp. This movement wants some care, if done with both hands.

(v.) The grasp may be changed while in a momentary handstand.

(vi.) After a drop back from the rest you may change the grasp with one hand or both, and you may change the grasp in the same way after a drop back from the side seat or riding seat, and bringing the leg or legs in front of the bar. As I have explained, when you do a drop back the legs will leave the bar, and then, if you wish to continue, they must be brought back again; the moment for the change is when the legs have just left the bar; these changes, if made with both hands, require care at first.

§ 326. The following exercises will serve to illustrate the changes of grasp described in the last paragraph—

(i.) Hang, Swing, Pass Both Legs Between Hands, Half Free Seat Circle Forwards to Side Seat, Change to Reverse Grasp, Clear Seat Circle Forwards to Side Seat, Change to Ordinary Grasp, Drop Back, Bring Legs in Front of Bar, Swing Back, Change Right Hand to Reverse Grasp, Swing Forward, Upstart, Change Left Hand to Reverse Grasp, Front Circle, Change Bôth Hands to Ordinary Grasp, Short Circle, Drop Back, and Short Underswing to Ground.

(ii.) Hang with Reverse Grasp, Back-Up, Change to Ordinary Grasp, Short Circle, Drop Back, Change Right Hand to Reverse Grasp, Bring Right Leg Between Hands, Half Mill Circle Forwards, Half Right Circle with Left Leg, changing Left Hand to Reverse Grasp, and Clear Seat Circle Forwards to Ground.

(iii.) From the Rest, Drop Back, Change to Reverse Grasp, Upstart, Change to Ordinary Grasp, Front Circle, Change to Reverse Grasp, Short Underswing, Change to Ordinary Grasp, Bring Both Legs Between Hands, and Half Free Seat Circle Forwards to Ground.

(iv.) Hang with Reverse Grasp, Take a Slight Swing, Clear Circle to Handstand, Change to Ordinary Grasp, Long Circle Backwards, Half Long Circle Backwards to Free Rest, Drop Back, and Short Underswing to Ground.

(v.) Hang with Reverse Grasp, Take a Slight Swing, Back-Up to Handstand, Long Circle Forwards to Handstand, Change Grasp, Long Circle Backwards, Short Circle to Handstand, Half Long Circle Backwards to Free Rest, Short Circle to Free Rest, Half Right Circle with Both Legs, Free Seat Circle Backwards, Drop Back, and Short Underswing to Ground.

TURNS.

§ 327. Great variety may be introduced into exercises by means of turns. You must remember that what was in front of the bar before you turn, becomes behind the bar after a turn, therefore, in discussing the turns, it is necessary to explain whether you reckon from the original or ultimate position.

§ 328. *Turns in the Hang with a Swing in Front of Bar* (*reckoning from the original position*).

(i.) Swing with the right hand in ordinary grasp, and at the forward extremity of the swing let go with the left hand, do a half right turn and take hold of the bar again and swing forward. You may take hold of the bar with the left hand in either ordinary or reverse grasp, and will have accordingly either combined or reverse grasp for your forward swing.

(ii.) Swing with right hand in reverse grasp, and at the forward extremity of the swing let go with the left hand, do a half left turn, take hold of the bar again with the left hand and swing forward. You may take hold of the bar with the left hand in either ordinary or reverse grasp, and you will then have accordingly either ordinary or combined grasp. This movement is much easier if you start with the left hand in ordinary grasp, than if you take a reverse grasp with both hands.

(iii.) Swing with ordinary grasp, and at the forward extremity of the swing let go with both hands, do a half turn in the air and catch hold of the bar again.

In all these turns, the main difficulties are, to keep the legs together, and to avoid having a swing sideways on the return swing. At first your legs are certain to open wide, and you are equally certain to be quite unconscious of the fact.

§ 329. *Turns in the Hang with a Swing Behind the Bar* (*reckoning from the original position*).

(i.) Swing with the right hand in ordinary grasp, and at the back end of your swing let go with the left hand and do a half right turn, take hold of the bar again with the left hand and swing back. You will, of course, have a reverse grasp with the right hand, and may have either grasp with the left hand.

(ii.) Swing with the right hand in reverse grasp, and at the back end of the swing let go with the left hand and do a half left turn, take hold of the bar again with the left hand and swing back. You will, of course, have an ordinary grasp with the right hand, and may have either grasp with the left hand.

These turns are in themselves very constrained and awkward movements. However, while doing either of these turns, you may raise the feet to the bar and do an upstart on the return swing, and these movements are very pretty.

§ 330. *Turns in the Hang, bringing Feet to Bar.*

(i.) Hang with the right hand in ordinary grasp, take a swing, let go with left hand as you take the swing, and do a half right turn, grasp with the left hand again and swing forwards. Start as if you were going to take a swing, as described in § 287, but, as you throw the body and legs out, let go with the left hand, do a half right turn, take hold with the left hand again in ordinary grasp, and swing forwards; you will now have combined grasp. It is possible to get a very good swing in this way.

(ii.) Hang with right hand in reverse grasp, take a swing, let go with left hand as you take the swing, and do a half left turn, grasp with the left hand again and swing forwards. This is done in a similar manner to the last exercise. It is very difficult.

(iii.) Hang, take a swing, leg go with both hands as you take the swing, and do a half left turn, grasp the bar and swing forwards. This is done in a similar manner to the last exercise, and is also difficult.

§ 331. *Turns from the Drop Back from the Rest.*

(i.) Drop back from the rest, throw the body up, let go with the left hand, do a half right turn, grasp with the left hand and swing forwards. This is just like exercise (i.), described in the last paragraph.

(ii.) Drop back from the rest, throw the body up, let go with both hands, do a half turn, grasp the bar again and swing forwards. This is just like exercise (iii.), described in the last paragraph.

§ 332. *The Giant Back-Up.*

' (i.) Hang, Swing, and Giant Back-Up with Half Right Turn on Right Arm. Hang, swing, and, as you approach the forward extremity of your swing, let go with the left hand and do a half right turn and replace the left hand, at the same time rising above the bar so that you come to the rest or free rest. You will, of course, have the right hand reversed; you may take which grasp you please with the left hand. This exercise requires a very good swing, and is accordingly most easily done after a long underswing from the rest. It may be followed by a vault left; or by a front circle, short circle, or drop back, with or without a change of grasp of the right hand. If you do this giant back-up after a long underswing from the handstand and turn late, you may even come to the handstand, and, if you then take reverse grasp with the left hand, you may continue with the long circle forwards, and in this way long circles backwards may be followed by long circles forwards in the same direction. This change from the long circle backwards to the long circle forwards is one of the finest movements which can be done on the bar. This giant back-up may also be followed by a leg circle. It might perhaps be followed by a squatting or straddling movement, but I have never seen these combinations accomplished. '

(ii.) Hang, with Combined Grasp, Right Hand Reversed, Swing, and Giant Back-Up with Half Left Turn on Right Arm. Hang, swing, and, as you approach the forward end of your swing, let go with the left hand and do a half left turn and replace the left hand, at the same time rising above the bar and coming to a rest or free rest. You will, of course, have the right hand in ordinary grasp ; you may take which grasp you please with the left hand. This giant back-up may be followed by a short circle or drop back ; it might perhaps be followed by a vault, leg circle, or squatting or straddling movement, or by a front circle, but I have never seen these combinations accomplished. It is extremely difficult to do the exercise at all.

§ 333. *From the Rest, Drop Back and Half Right Turn on Right Arm, Rising in Front of Bar (reckoning from original 'position) to Rest.* Proceed as in exercise (i.) in § 331, but, instead of dropping back as if you intended to do a short upstart, drop back with much less bend at the waist, as if you intended to do a short circle, and turn rather late, at the same time rising above the bar. This exercise is of extreme difficulty ; it may be followed by vault or leg circle, or by a short circle or drop back with or without changing the grasp of the right hand. I have seen this exercise done to the handstand with a movement somewhat similar to that made in doing a giant back-up to the handstand, as described in the last paragraph.

§ 334. *Turns in the Rest.*
(i.) From the Rest, Let go Left Hand and Half Left Turn to Back Rest. This is an obvious movement and hardly requires description ; it is, however, very often difficult to do from a free rest with pause. It may be done after an upstart, front circle, or back-up, and you may continue with a forward seat circle or a hand circle. It may also be done

M

after a short circle, but you must begin your turn in that case before you finish the circle ; this combination is very pretty.

(ii.) From the Rest, Let go Both Hands and Half Turn to Side Seat. This is comparatively easy, and may be done from a free rest after an upstart, front circle, or back-up. It is most easily followed by a seat circle or half seat circle backwards.

§ 335. *Turns in the Back Rest.*

From the Back Rest with Reverse Grasp Let go Left Hand and Half Right Turn to Rest or Free Rest. This is an obvious movement, it may be done to a free rest ; for example, after a free seat circle forwards, and you may continue with a short circle or drop back. To accomplish this movement, you must begin to turn rather before you finish the seat circle.

§ 336. You may turn in the riding rest very easily, either letting go one hand or both, and these turns are rather effective if done without any pause while passing through the position.

§ 337. You may turn from the back rest or straddle rest, dropping below the bar as you turn, and continuing with a drop back or long underswing. This turn is very effective after a half free seat circle forwards with the legs astride the arms.

§ 338. You may combine leg circles with turns, doing exercises very like those on the horse, which enable you to change from the saddle to the croup, and *vice versâ*. For example—

(i.) From the Rest with Right Hand Reversed, Half Right Circle with Both Legs, and, Without Replacing Left Hand, Half Right Turn to Free Rest to the Original Right of the Right Hand. This is like the turn to the front rest on the croup, mentioned in § 95.

(ii.) From the Rest with Right Hand Reversed, Half Right Circle with Both Legs, and, Without Replacing Left Hand, Half Right Circle with One Leg over Bar to Original Right of Right Hand, coming to Side Riding Rest. These exercises are like those described in §§ 85, 86.

(iii.) From the Rest with Right Hand Reversed, Half Right Circle with Both Legs, and, Without Replacing Left Hand, Half Right Circle with Both Legs over Bar to Original Right of Right Hand, coming to Back Rest or to Ground behind Bar (reckoning from the original position). These exercises are like those described in § 88.

(iv.) From Side Riding Rest with Right Leg Forward and Right Hand Reversed, Half Right Circle with Left Leg, and, Without Replacing Left Hand, Half Right Circle with Left Leg over Bar to Original Right of Right Hand, coming to Riding Rest.

The exercises (i.), (ii.), (iii.), may be done after an upstart or front circle, but these combinations are extremely difficult; they may also, on a low bar, be done from the ground.

§ 339. *Turns in the Handstand.* From the handstand, with the right hand in ordinary grasp, you may do a half right turn on the right arm and come to a handstand with the right hand in reverse grasp. I have never seen this turn done in a stationary handstand, but the giant back-up to the handstand, described in § 332, and the drop back and half right turn, rising to the handstand, described in § 333, really introduce this turn, in the one case after a long circle backwards, and in the other case after a short circle to the handstand. Again, from the handstand with the right hand in reverse grasp, you may do a half left turn on the right arm and come to a handstand with the right hand in ordinary grasp. This turn may be done after a forward long circle, and you may continue with a long circle backwards. In this way, alternating half right and half left turns in the handstand, you may do alternate forward and backward long circles in the same direction. Again, after a long circle backwards, if you just overbalance forward, you may change the grasp of the right hand and then do this turn, and continue with a long circle backwards in the opposite direction.

§ 340. The following exercises introduce turns—

(i.) On a Low Bar, From the Stand with Combined Grasp, Right Hand Reversed, Long Underswing, Pass Right Leg Between Arms, Half Free Mill Circle Forwards, Half Right Circle with Left Leg, and, Without Replacing Left Hand, Half Right Turn on Right Arm to Free Rest, Short Circle, Drop Back, Bring Legs behind Bar Astride Arms, Half Free Seat Circle Forwards, Pass over Bar with Half Left Turn letting go Both Hands (see § 337), Drop Back, Pass Right Leg between Arms, Half Free Mill Circle Forwards, Half Left Turn, Drop Back, and Short Underswing to Ground. This is an exercise of moderate difficulty.

(ii.) Hang with Combined Grasp, Right Hand Reversed, Swing, At Back End of Swing Half Left Turn on Right Arm and Upstart (see § 329), Half Left Turn to Back Rest, Drop Back, Upstart, Short Circle, Long Underswing, At Forward End of Swing Half Right Turn letting go Both Hands, Half Long Circle Backwards to Free Rest, Short Upstart, Front Circle, Throw up to Handstand, and High Front Vault Left. This is an exercise of considerable difficulty.

(iii.) Jump to Bar and Take a Swing with Half Left Turn on Left Arm, Taking Ordinary Grasp with Right Hand (see § 330), Giant Back-Up with Half Right Turn on Left Arm, Short Circle, Long Underswing, and Giant Back-Up

·with Half Right Turn on Right Arm, and Front Vault Left to Ground. This is an exercise of great difficulty.

(iv.) On a Low Bar, From Stand With Combined Grasp, Right Hand Reversed, Short Upstart, Half Right Circle with Both Legs, and, Without Replacing Left Hand, Half Right Turn to Free Rest, Short Circle, Half Left Turn to Free Back Rest, Free Seat Circle Forwards, Half Right Turn to Free Rest, Short Circle to Momentary Handstand, and Alight behind Bar with a Half Turn. This is an exercise of very great difficulty.

EXERCISES IN BACK HANG.

§ 341. *Swinging in Back Hang.* You may obtain a swing in the back hang from a back hang with the feet or thighs to the bar by throwing the legs from that position as far behind the bar as you can, and then letting them drop. This you may do with ordinary, combined, or reverse grasp. You may obtain a swing in the back hang in this manner after dropping back from a back rest, or after passing the feet through the hands after a forward swing, or a drop back, in the ordinary hang. You may also obtain a swing in the back hang with reverse grasp from the back rest by throwing the legs forward and dropping in front of the bar. In obtaining a swing in the back hang in the manner last explained, you must take your grasp with the hands rather closer together than usual, and be very careful to keep the arms perfectly straight, or you may come to the hang with a jerk, which will wrench the shoulders badly. You may obtain a swing in the back hang in this manner after squatting between the arms, or after a free seat circle forwards; but these combinations are very difficult.

§ 342. *Swing in Back Hang, and Circle Behind Bar to Back Rest.* As you swing backwards in the back hang, raise the legs, at the same time hollowing the back, and do a circle behind the bar to the back rest. You may do this with ordinary, combined, or reverse grasp, after a swing taken from the back hang with feet or thighs to the bar, or, with reverse grasp, after dropping in front of bar from the back rest. This last movement is a sort of half long circle forwards in the back hang, and is very effective.

§ 343. *Swing in Back Hang, and Long Back Upstart.* As you swing backwards in the back hang, hollow the back and raise the legs till you reach a horizontal position, then slightly bend the waist, and, as you begin to swing forwards again, hollow the back very sharply, and rise in front of the bar to the back rest. This exercise is most easily done with reverse grasp after dropping from the back rest in front of the bar to the swing; it may also be done after obtaining the swing by passing the feet between the hands from a swing in ordinary hang, and in this manner it may be done with ordinary, combined, or reverse grasp.

§ 344. *From the Back Rest with Reverse Grasp, Short Back Upstart.* From the back rest, begin as if you intended to do a free seat circle forwards with a hollow back, as described in § 263, but, instead of circling the bar, reach a momentary back lever, and then return in front of the bar to the back rest again.

§ 345. *From the Side Seat, Take Reverse Grasp with the Hands Wide Apart, Drop in Front of Bar, Dislocate, and Back-Up with Twisted Grasp, Let Go, Take Ordinary Grasp, and Short Circle, continuing as you please.* In the side seat, take a reverse grasp with the hands very wide apart, throw the legs and body as far to the front as you can, drop boldly, and, as you pass under the bar, dislocate, coming, of course, to an ordinary hang with twisted grasp, continue the swing, and do a back-up, as you rise above the bar, let go, and replace the hands on the bar with ordinary grasp, and do a short circle. · This movement is very effective, and not so difficult as it looks; you must be very careful to keep the arms absolutely straight till after the dislocation, or else you may wrench the shoulders badly.

MISCELLANEOUS EXERCISES.

§ 346. There are a number of circles on the bar something like seat or knee circles which I may mention. They may all be done with the legs between the hands, or the hands between the legs, or with one leg between the hands and one outside; in the forward circles you must take reverse grasp, and in the backward circles ordinary grasp.

(i.) *Feet Circles.* In these circles you hold the bar with the hands, and place the soles of the feet against the bar; you may do these circles forwards or backwards. They are ungainly movements at the best, and not particularly difficult.

(ii.) *Instep Circles with Bent Knees.* In these circles you hold the bar with the hands, and place the insteps against the bar; when above the bar you are almost kneeling on the bar, but you have the bar against the insteps, and not against the shins. You may do these circles forwards or backwards.

(iii.) *Forward Instep Circles with Straight Legs.* In these circles the knees are straight and the feet hooked round the bar. The easiest is with the legs outside the hands. Come to the front rest with reverse grasp, raise the hips, straddling the legs till the front of the insteps are against the bar, then circle forwards; as you rise to the rest again the feet will leave the bar. Circles of this kind, with the feet, or one foot, between the hands, require exceptional suppleness.

§ 347. Knee circles and seat circles on the knees may be done holding the bar with one hand only. There are sixteen possible knee circles of this kind on the right knee, and twelve possible seat circles of this kind with the right hand, as you will find if you ring the changes. Some of these are, however, extremely difficult. Knee circles and seat circles on the knees may also be done with crossed arms with one or both legs between the arms, and these movements admit of some variety.

§ 348. Circles somewhat similar to knee circles may be done clasping the hands round the knee which is hooked round the bar, so that the bar is between the knee and the arms. Similar circles may be done with both knees hooked round the bar with the arms clasping one knee or both knees. These circles may be done forwards or backwards, but they are ungainly movements.

§ 349. *Knee and Instep Circles.* From the side riding seat with the left leg forward, grasp the bar to the left of the left leg with left hand at some distance from the leg, pass the right leg to the right, and hook the toe of the right foot round the bar, pass the hips a little to the rear, and raise them a little, and hook the left knee round the bar, then throw the right hand out at right angles to the body, and circle the bar in this position. You may do the circle forwards or backwards, and either way with either grasp of the left hand. The easiest circle is the forward circle with left hand in reverse grasp. These circles are rather effective movements.

§ 350. *Circle with Toe of One Foot on Bar.* From the rest with combined grasp, right hand reversed, pass the right leg over the bar to the left of the hands, let the arms bend, and slide the right leg to the left, carry the left leg to the left, and hook the toe of the left foot round the bar, then let the left elbow sink below the bar, and at the same time let the hips sink below the bar in front of it, so that you are supported by the hands and the toe of the left foot alone, with the right elbow above the bar, and the left elbow below it, the back being hollow, and the body close to the bar, and parallel to it; then circle the bar forwards in this position.

§ 351. *Hock Hang, Swing, and Circles.* You may hang from the bar from the hocks with the knees hooked over the bar without touching the bar with the hands, and in this position you may swing; if you take a moderate swing, and, just before you reach the forward extremity of the swing, straighten the knees, you will alight on the ground. If you take a good swing you may rise in front of the bar or behind the bar, coming to the side seat. From the side seat, you may drop behind the bar, without touching the bar with the hands, to the hock hang, and, if you drop boldly with a good swing, you may in this manner circle the bar completely, and return to the side seat. It is worth while learning these swings and circles, although there is not the slightest difficulty in them, because they may help you to avoid a fall, and they also may be introduced rather neatly into combinations. You may do a hock circle hanging from one hock alone with the legs astride the bar. If you have the right knee over the bar, and hook the left knee round the right ankle, it is possible to do a hock circle forwards in this way. These movements, however, are ungainly, and of little use.

§ 352. There are a few exercises on the bar which are more fit for acrobats than for gymnasts, but which I ought perhaps to mention, although I do not recommend your attempting them.

(i.) *The Backaway.* As you swing forward in a backward long circle, and just after you have passed the vertical position below the bar, let go, do a back somersault, and alight. The back should be hollow throughout the movement. A backaway may be done with a double somersault, and I believe the back may be kept hollow even in this movement.

(ii.) *The Frontaway.* Take as good a swing as you can, and, as you approach the back end of your swing, let go, do a front somersault, and alight. This exercise might perhaps be done, after a forward long circle, with a hollow back; but I have always seen it done with the ordinary grasp, and the body bent at the waist, and, of course, done in this way it is an ungainly movement.

(iii.) *Drop Back, and Front Somersault.* After a drop back, let go the bar, as if you intended to do an ordinary short underswing to the ground, but with a more vigorous effort, and, when you let go, do a front somersault. This is rather effective; I do not know whether it is difficult.

(iv.) *Somersaults from a Standing Position on the Bar.* You may stand on the bar and do a back somersault, alighting either in front of the bar or behind it. You may also do a front somersault alighting in front of the bar. I do not think I ever saw a front somersault done alighting behind the bar, but perhaps it is possible.

(v.) *Somersault from Hock Swing.* In the course of a hock swing you may reach a position in which the body is behind the bar and a little above it; from this position you may, with a kick, raise the knees from the bar, and do a back somersault, alighting behind the bar.

(vi.) *Slip Out from Hock Swing.* As you swing backwards in a hock swing, you may unhook the knees and let the legs slide over the bar, and alight behind it.

(vii.) *Still Drop from Hock Hang.* From a hock hang,

with the body perfectly still, you may let go with the knees, and, with a sudden jerk, alight on the feet.

(viii.) *Flip Off.* From a side seat, you may let the body fall backwards, and then bring the feet over the head, and alight behind the bar. A similar movement may be done from a position in which you lie across the bar resting on the hollow of the back.

There are no doubt many other acrobatic performances possible, but the list I have given includes all those commonly done.

CHAPTER IV.

PARALLEL BARS.

PART I.—*PRELIMINARY.*

§§ 353–357. Apparatus and General Definitions—§§ 358–
367. Positions and Grasp.

APPARATUS AND GENERAL DEFINITIONS.

§ 353. The parallel bars may conveniently be about
7 ft. 6 in. in length, but the exact length is of no great
importance; the ends of the bars should project at least
a foot beyond the uprights. The bars should be high enough
to allow your feet to be just clear of the ground when
you are in the upper arm rest (see § 366) with the toes
pointed. The clear distance between the bars should be
just sufficient to allow you to drop back between the bars,
as described in § 493, if you keep the arms perfectly
straight, and bring the shoulders well forward; 17½ in.
will be found a fair average distance. It is most important
that the parallel bars should be perfectly firm, so that they
will not shift or tip up; accordingly, either the uprights
and feet should be extremely heavy, or the bars should be
fixed to the floor.

§ 354. *Cross and Side Positions.* Positions on the
parallel bars are divided into cross and side positions; in
cross positions, the shoulders are at right angles to the bars;
and, in side positions, the shoulders are parallel to the bars.

§ 355. *Meaning of "Right" and "Left" Bar, and of "Near" and "Off" Bar.* In any cross position, the bars are called respectively the "right" bar and the "left" bar, the left bar being to the left of the right bar from your point of view in that position. Thus, if you are between the bars, the right bar is on your right, and the left on your left. If you are outside the bars with the bars on your left, the nearer bar is the right bar. Observe that, if you turn round, the right bar becomes the left, and *vice versâ*. In any side position the bars are called respectively the "near" bar and the "off" bar, the off bar being in front of the near bar, so that if from a side position, with the body upright, you do a quarter right turn, the off bar will become the left bar, and the near bar will become the right bar. In the description of exercises begun from a cross position, and involving turns, however, it is often convenient to continue to distinguish the bars as right and left, although you may have reached a side position. Similarly in the description of exercises begun from a side position, and involving turns, it is often convenient to continue to distinguish the bars as off and near, although you may have reached a cross position.

§ 356. *Meaning of "Forwards," "Backwards," "In Front," "Behind."* If you are in a cross position with the head up, the direction in which you are looking is "forwards," and the opposite direction "backwards;" and these directions retain these names so long as you do not turn to the right or left. If you are head downwards, therefore, in a cross position, *e.g.* in a shoulderstand (see §§ 385, 386), you are considered to be looking backwards. Any point is said to be in front of any other if you have to move forwards from the latter to the former, and, of course, the latter point is behind the former. Accordingly, if you are head downwards in a cross position, the back of your head is considered to be in front of your face.

§ 357. *Meaning of " Near End " and " Further End" of Bars*. In cross positions the end of the bars furthest forward is called the "further end ;" the other end is called the "near end."

POSITIONS AND GRASP.

§ 358. *General Rules*. Positions in which the weight is entirely supported on one bar are described exactly in the same way as similar positions on the horizontal bar, but it is, of course, necessary to state on which bar the weight is to be supported. Positions in which the weight is partly supported on one bar and partly on the other may often be described as positions on the one bar with one or both hands, or one or both legs on the other bar. For example, if you come to a cross riding seat on the right bar, and place the left hand on the left bar, your position may be described as a "cross riding seat on right bar with left hand on left bar." In the description of positions on the parallel bars, however, which are not described with reference to one bar in the manner just explained, it is assumed, so far as nothing to the contrary appears—

(i.) That the position is to be a cross, and not a side, position.

(ii.) That the right bar is to be grasped by the right hand, and the left bar by the left hand, with the hands opposite each other, so that the straight line joining them is at right angles to the bars.

(iii.) That the arms are to be straight, and, if the arms are directed to be bent, that they are, unless further directions are given, to be bent as much as possible.

(iv.) That the legs are to be straight, and closed, and are

to hang vertically downwards, or as nearly vertically downwards as possible under the circumstances, and that, if the position of one leg is given, the other is to be straight, and to hang vertically downwards, or as nearly vertically downwards as possible under the circumstances.

(v.) That the body is to be upright, or as nearly upright as possible.

You must be careful to apply these rules only so far as nothing to the contrary appears. If two of these rules in any particular portion contradict each other, the earlier rule is to be followed.

§ 359. *The Hang.* The word "hang" is used in the same sense as in the description of positions on the horizontal bar; hangs on one bar alone are, of course, described exactly like hangs on the horizontal bar. In a hang from both bars there are, as a rule, three possible grasps for each hand; first, with the palm of the hand turned towards the other bar when the hand is said to have the "outside grasp;" secondly, with the palm of the hand turned away from the other bar, the right hand being turned to the left, or the left to the right, when the hand is said to have an "inside grasp;" thirdly, with the palm of the hand turned away from the other bar, the right hand being turned to the right, or the left to the left, when the hand is said to have the "reverse grasp." If you come to a side hang on the off bar, and do a quarter left turn, letting go with the left hand, and take hold of the left bar with the left hand, you will have an inside grasp with the right hand, if you had ordinary grasp originally; an outside grasp, if you had reverse grasp originally. There are other possible grasps at the ends of the bars. At the near end of the bars you may take a grasp intermediate between an inside and outside grasp, with the hands on the bars, and the wrists over the ends, so that the ends of the bars are against the front of the forearms just above the wrists. Secondly, at the further ends of the bars, you may take a grasp intermediate between an outside and a reverse grasp, so that the wrists are over the ends of the bars. Cross hangs on both bars, like hangs on a horizontal bar, are divided into ordinary and back hangs; unless the contrary appears in the description of a cross hang on both bars, you are intended to be in an ordinary hang, as distinguished from a back hang. I may point out that, in accordance with the rules given in § 358, the word "hang" alone means an ordinary cross hang with one hand on each bar. It remains, of course, to state the grasp, and practically also the position of the legs, which cannot hang straight down, except on an unusually high pair of bars.

§ 360. *Seats.* Seats on one bar alone are, of course, described exactly like seats on the horizontal bar. The only seats of any practical use on both bars are the riding seat and the side riding seat. The riding seat is shown in Fig. 18. It is not easy at first to come to the proper position in the riding seat, as there is a considerable strain on the thighs; in the riding seat, you should turn the knees somewhat in so as to grasp the bars with the inside of the thighs. The side riding seat you may reach from the riding seat, by doing a quarter turn; it is like the side riding seat on the horse. I may point out that the expressions "riding seat" and "side riding seat" used alone mean respectively, in accordance with the rules given, the riding seat and the side riding seat on both bars.

§ 361. *Leaning Hangs.* The expression "leaning hang" has the same meaning as in the description of positions on the horizontal bar.

§ 362. *Rests.* The word "rest" has the same general

meaning as in the description of positions on the horizontal
bar. Rests on one bar alone are, of course, described

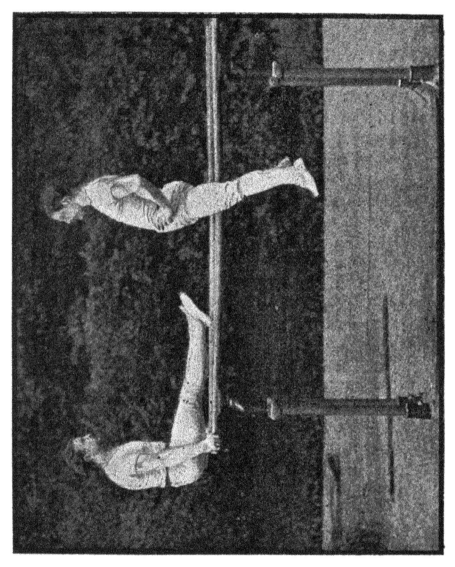

Fig. 18.—RIDING SEAT AND HALF LEVER.

exactly like rests on the horizontal bar. So far, however,
as nothing to the contrary appears, the expression rest, in

N

accordance with the rules given, means a cross rest with one hand on each bar. These rests are of great variety, and are further discussed in the next paragraph.

§ 363. *Cross Rests with One Hand on Each Bar.* In a cross rest with one hand on each bar, there are three possible grasps for each hand; first, with the palm of the hand towards the other bar, when the hand is said to have "ordinary grasp;" secondly, with the palm of the hand turned away from the other bar, the left hand being turned to the right, and the right hand to the left, when the hand is said to have the "reverse grasp;" thirdly, with the palm of the hand turned away from the other bar, the left hand being turned to the left, and the right hand to the right, when the hand is said to have the "twisted grasp." If nothing to the contrary appears in the description of a rest, you are intended to have the ordinary grasp with both hands. The reverse and twisted grasps are of little importance. The following are the most important positions among the cross rests with one hand on each bar; some of them have special short names—

(i.) *The Rest.* This, in accordance with the rules given, means a position in which the arms are straight and the body and legs vertical. In this position you must have the back perfectly hollow, the head up, the chin well pressed back, and the shoulders pressed down. Beginners are apt, in the rest, to let the weight down between the shoulders, so that the shoulders are up about their ears.

(ii.) *The Bent Arm Rest.* You may reach this position from the rest by letting the elbows bend as far as you can consistently with good style. In the bent arm rest, you must keep the back hollow, the head up, and the chin well pressed back. Beginners are apt to bend at the waist, and let the head drop forward; this arises partly from getting too low.

(iii.) *The Half Lever.* This is a short name for "rest with legs in half lever." You may reach it from the rest by raising the legs till they are horizontal. This position is of fundamental importance on the parallel bars, and is shown in Fig. 18. The tendency at first is to get the hips too far back, so that you have to bend too much at the waist in order to get the legs horizontal. You may take it that it is almost impossible to get the legs too far forward in this position.

(iv.) *The Riding Rest, Hands in Front.* This is a short name for "rest with legs in riding seat behind hands." You may reach this position from the riding seat on both bars, by taking hold of the bars in front of the body and leaning slightly forward, letting a share of your weight come on the hands, taking care to keep the back perfectly hollow.

(v.) *The Riding Rest, Hands Behind.* This is a short name for "rest with legs in riding seat in front of hands." You may reach this position from the riding seat on both bars by taking hold of the bars behind the body and leaning slightly back, letting a share of your weight come on the hands. In slow exercises, where you have to retain this position for a certain time, you should hollow the back as nearly as you can, but where you merely reach the position momentarily this is not necessary.

(vi.) *The Outside Rest in Front of Right Hand.* This is a short name for " rest with legs over right bar in front of right hand." You may reach this position from a side seat on the off bar by placing the right hand on the off bar to the right of the legs, and the left hand on the near bar opposite the right hand, turning the shoulders a quarter turn to the left, and turning the hips a little to the left. In the position the seat, not the thighs, should be in contact with the bar, the back should be nearly hollow, and the feet rather in front of the hips.

(vii.) *The Outside Rest Behind Right Hand.* This is a short name for "rest with legs over right bar behind right hand." You may reach this position from the side seat on the off bar by placing the right hand on the off bar to the left of the legs, and the left hand on the near bar opposite the right hand, at the same time turning the shoulders nearly a quarter turn to the left, turning the hips slightly to the left and letting the feet come rather forward. There is another variation of this position in which you turn the hips through a quarter turn and rest on the outside of the left thigh. In describing this position, the words "legs in cross seat," must be added, so that the description of the position is, "outside rest behind right hand with legs in cross seat."

(viii.) *Rest with Legs over Right Bar Astride Right Arm.* This position requires no further explanation.

(ix., x.) *Rest with Legs in Riding Seat on Right Bar in Front of or Behind Right Hand.* These positions require no further explanation.

(xi.) *Rest with Left Leg over Right Bar in Front of Right Hand.* You may reach this position from the rest by carrying the left leg over the right bar in front of the right hand, and resting most of the weight on the outside of the left thigh, letting the right leg hang straight down.

(xii.) *Rest with Left Leg over Right Bar in Front of Right Hand and under Right Leg.* To reach this position you may come to the outside rest in front of the right hand, and then turn the hips to the left and carry the right leg over the bar, so that the bar is between the legs, and the outside of the left thigh rests against the bar.

(xiii.) *Rest with Left Leg over Right Bar Behind Right*

Hand and under Right Leg. You may reach this position from No. xi., described above, by letting go with the right hand and placing it in front of the legs, and shifting the left hand forward till it is opposite the right hand.

(xiv.) *Rest with Left Leg over Right Bar Behind Right Hand and over Right Leg.* You may reach this position from No. xii., described above, by letting go with the right hand and placing it in front of the legs, and shifting the left hand forward till it is opposite the right hand.

(xv.) *Back Leaning Rest.* This is a short name for " rest with feet on bars in front of hands." You support the weight on the hands and feet, with one foot on each bar, resting on the outside of the instep, and with the back as nearly hollow as possible.

(xvi.) *Front Leaning Rest.* This is a short name for " rest with feet on bars behind hands." You support the weight on the hands and feet, with one foot on each bar, resting on the inside of the insteps, and with the back hollow.

§ 364. *Rests with Both Hands on one Bar.* The principal rests with both hands on one bar are—

(i.) *Front Rest on Off Bar with One Leg, or Both Legs, over Near Bar.* You may reach these positions respectively from a side riding rest or front rest on the near bar by shifting the hands on to the off bar, keeping the back hollow.

(ii.) *Back Rest on Near Bar with One Leg, or Both Legs, over Off Bar.* You may reach these positions respectively from a side riding seat or side seat on the off bar by shifting the hand on to the near bar, and leaning back.

§ 365. *Forearm Rests.* You may support your weight on the bars wholly or partly on the forearms, grasping the bars with the hands, and letting the forearms rest on the top of the bars. These positions are called " forearm rests." They are not of very great importance.

§ 366. *Upper Arm Rests.* In these positions the weight is supported wholly or mainly on the upper arms. If from

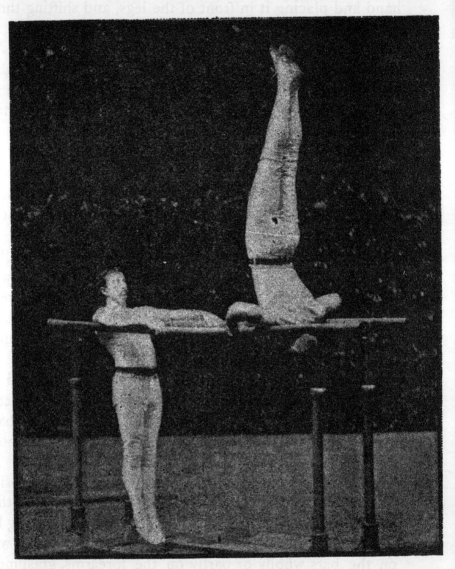

Fig. 19.—UPPER ARM REST AND DOUBLE SHOULDERSTAND.

a cross stand between the bars you place the arms over the bars, at right angles to them, and raise the weight on the arms so that you are supported on the upper arms with the bars close to the arm-pits, the position you reach is called the "upper arm rest without hands." If from this position you bring the hands forwards and grasp the bars, with the arms very slightly bent, and the elbows just outside the bars, you reach the "upper arm rest," which is shown in Fig. 19. This position is of great importance; you must get the shoulders and elbows well down, so that the head is as high as possible. If from the upper arm rest without hands you pass the hands backwards and place them on the bars, you reach the "upper arm rest with hands behind." In this position you should, in the absence of further directions, let the hands rest on the bars, with the fingers outside and the thumbs inside the bars, but without grasping the bars.

§ 367. *Other Positions.* There are other positions on the bars of great importance, which will be discussed in the course of the chapter; among these the most important are handstands, shoulderstands, the front lever in the rest, and elbow levers.

PART II.—*SLOW EXERCISES.*

§ 368. Exercises in Hang—§§ 369–377. Exercises in Rest —§§ 378–382. Exercises Leading from Hang to Rest, and *vice versâ*—§§ 383, 384. Exercises in Upper Arm Rest—§§ 385–397. Exercises Combining Rests and Upper Arm Rests with Shoulderstands, Handstands, etc.—§§ 398–409. Exercises in Handstand and Shoulderstand—§§ 410–420. Elbow Levers.

EXERCISES IN HANG.

§ 368. There are hardly any slow exercises in the hang

on the parallel bars at all peculiar to the instrument; you may, of course, do a number of the slow exercises in a cross hang between the parallel bars which you may do on a horizontal bar in a side hang. You may also do slow exercises in the side hang on one bar and combine them with slow exercises in the cross hang on both bars; but none of these exercises require particular description.

EXERCISES IN REST.

§ 369. *From the Rest, Sink to Bent Arm Rest, Rise again to Rest.* This exercise calls for no further description; you must be very careful to keep the head well up, with the chin pressed back, and to keep the back perfectly hollow.

§ 370. *Travels in the Rest.* You may "travel," that is, move along the bars, in the rest in several ways—

(i.) You may travel either forwards or backwards, moving the hands alternately; that is, raising each hand in turn, and moving it a few inches along its own bar. In these movements you must endeavour to let the body move steadily without any swing either forwards, backwards, or sideways, and to take the steps with the hands in even time without pause between the steps.

(ii.) You may travel either forwards or backwards, moving both hands together; that is, with a series of jumps from the hands. In these movements you must keep the arms perfectly straight, and the back hollow, and avoid any sort of swing. The jump is accomplished by a movement of the shoulder; the tendency at first is to bend at the waist, and get the jump by a sort of kick with the legs; but this you must avoid.

(iii.) You may travel forwards or backwards, moving one

hand at a time, or both hands together, with the legs in various positions; for example, with one leg, or both legs, in the half lever. Travels with both legs in the half lever are of extreme difficulty.

§ 371. *Travels in Bent Arm Rest.* You may travel in the bent arm rest, in the same way as in a straight arm rest, either backwards or forwards, and raising the hands alternately, or both hands together. These movements are much easier than the travels in the straight arm rest to do well; the only difficulty is to keep the back perfectly hollow.

§ 372. *Lion Crawl.* From the bent arm rest, let go with the left hand, coming to a cross bent arm rest on the right arm alone, pass the left hand along the left bar, and grasp the bar again, rise to the rest, sink again to bent arm rest, and repeat the movement on the other side, and so on alternately right and left. You may do a lion crawl forwards or backwards, and you may do a lion crawl without rising to the rest at each step. You must be careful to keep the back perfectly hollow throughout the movement. In a lion crawl forwards, when you let go with the left hand, pass it first to the rear, and straighten the arm, then move it forwards close past your side with the arm perfectly straight, and do not bend it again until you have raised it above the bars in front of you. Similarly, in a lion crawl backwards, pass the hand backwards with a straight arm.

§ 373. *From the Rest, Come to Front Lever in the Rest.* From the rest, lean forward, and raise the legs behind you until you are horizontal. The front lever in the rest is not easy to retain; you must grasp the bars very loosely. The higher you can get the body, keeping it, of course, horizontal, the better. The front lever in the rest is shown in Fig. 20 ; but in the figure the feet are a good deal too high.

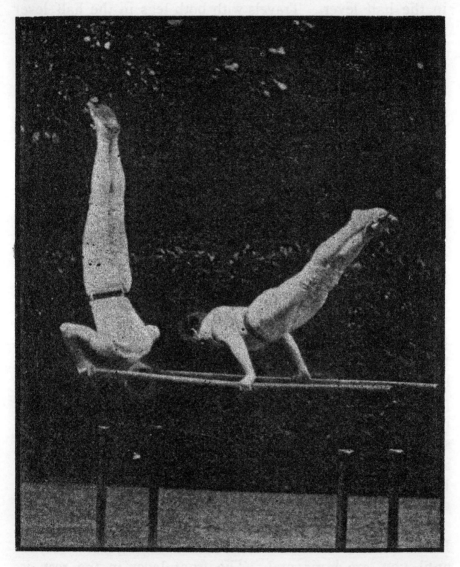

Fig. 20.—FRONT LEVER IN THE REST AND BENT ARM HANDSTAND.

§ 374. *From Riding Rest, Hands in Front, Come to Front Lever in the Rest.* From the rest mentioned, lean forward, getting all the weight on the hands, close the legs, and remain in the lever.

§ 375. You may do the exercise last described, then gradually come to the rest, raise the legs to half lever, straddle to the riding rest with hands behind, then shift the hands in front of the body, and repeat the movement. You may also do a similar exercise backwards. In these exercises you must be careful to show the riding seat quite distinctly while you are shifting the hands, with the back quite hollow, as explained in § 360.

§ 376. *From the Half Lever, Quarter Right Turn to Back Rest on Right Bar with Legs in Half Lever.* From the half lever, turn to the right, carrying the legs over the right bar, and shift the left hand on to the right bar, keeping the legs horizontal throughout the movement.

§ 377. You may do an exercise similar to that last described, returning from the one bar to the half lever on both. If you turn from both bars to one, and then further to the right, and return to the half lever on both bars, you have done a half turn, and the movement is described shortly as "half right turn with legs in half lever."

EXERCISES LEADING FROM HANG TO REST, AND VICE VERSA.

§ 378. *At Near End of Bars, Slow Rise to Rest.* Take the grasp, described in § 359, with the wrists over the ends of the bars, then do a slow rise, just as you would on a horizontal bar. If the bars are rather too wide it is possible to do a slow rise at the centre of the bars, starting with an inside grasp with the wrists raised above the bars. In this exercise you must let the elbows pass well to the rear as you rise; I have never seen this done on bars of the proper width.

§ 379. *At Further End of Bars, Slow ·Circle to Rest.* Take the grasp, described in § 359, with the wrists over the bars, and circle as you would on a horizontal bar. As the legs pass over the head you must let the hands slip round, supporting the weight on the wrists without grasping the bars, so that when you reach the rest you have the ordinary grasp.

§ 380. *At Further End of Bars, Slow Circle to Front Lever in Rest.* Proceed as in the exercise described in the last paragraph, but, instead of letting the legs sink to the rest as you finish the circle, remain in the lever.

§ 381. *From the Hang on Near Bar with Right Hand Reversed and Legs in Half Lever, Shear Mount to Riding Rest with Hands in Front.* From the hang mentioned, raise the feet between the bars, and pass them over the off bar, letting the left buttock come in contact with the off bar, then turn to the left, at the same time straddling the legs, bend the arms, and raise the right elbow above the bar (the movement of the arms is like that described in § 228), then let go with the left hand, continue turning to the left, rolling round on the left thigh, let the right thigh come in contact with the near bar, and place the left hand on the off bar.

§ 382. *From Front Leaning Rest, Sink to Hammock Hang, Rise again to Front Leaning Rest.* From the rest mentioned (No. xvi. in § 363), slide the feet somewhat backwards, and let the shoulders sink between the bars, so that you come to a back leaning hang with inside grasp, and with the feet on the bars (this leaning hang is called the "hammock hang"), then return to your original position. It is possible to do this exercise with straight arms, but it is much easier if you bend the arms as you pass between the bars.

EXERCISES IN UPPER ARM REST.

§ 383. In the upper arm rest it is possible to raise the body and legs forwards until you are horizontal; the position so reached is a "front lever in upper arm rest;" this position, however, requires exceptional strength to retain.

§ 384. In the upper arm rest, with hands behind, it is possible to raise the body and legs backwards till you are horizontal; the position so reached is a "back lever in upper arm rest with hands behind;" this position, however, requires exceptional strength to retain.

EXERCISES COMBINING RESTS AND UPPER ARM RESTS WITH SHOULDERSTANDS, HANDSTANDS, ETC.

§ 385. *From the Riding Rest, Hands in Front, Lift to Handstand with Bent Arms or to Double Shoulderstand.* In the riding rest, bring the legs rather forward, so that the thighs almost touch the hands, at the same time bending at the waist, then gradually get the whole weight on to the hands, raise the hips, bending the arms, and bending still more at the waist, till the hips are nearly above the head, then gradually hollow the back, and close the legs. The position you reach is called the handstand with bent arms, or bent arm handstand; it is shown in Fig. 20. This is, I think, the best way of trying to do a handstand at first; it requires a little more strength than to swing to a handstand, as explained in § 484; but, on the other hand, you reach the position slowly, and are less likely to get confused when you get there. At first you may keep the elbows close to the sides as you lift, so as to support some of your weight on them, and you may bend the knees; but afterwards you must learn to keep the knees perfectly straight, and the elbows quite clear of the body. If you reach the handstand with bent arms, and overbalance forwards, you should instantly move the elbows outwards, so that the upper arms are at right angles to the body; then the upper arms will come in contact with the bars, and you will find yourself in a position called "the double shoulderstand," which is shown in Fig. 19. This position is very easy to retain, as, of course, you are supported on a broad base. If in the double shoulderstand you overbalance forwards, bend at the waist, and bring the chin to the breast, so that you look at your toes, let go with the hands, roll round on the upper arms, and place the hands on the bars again in front of the shoulders; you then will be, or ought to be, in the second position shown in Fig. 21. However, at first you will be unable to get the hands on the bars until the legs have sunk considerably lower than the position there shown. Having placed the hands on the bars, let the feet drop till you come to the upper arm rest. It is important to become familiar with this method of rolling over from the bent arm handstand before you try any other exercises introducing handstands, because, when you are familiar with it, you will run no risk in learning these exercises. The movement is not at all difficult; but you should get help at first, because you may easily get confused and move the elbows in the wrong direction, so that you close them to the sides unintentionally, and slip through between the bars.

§ 386. *From the Riding Seat, Hands in Front, Lift to Shoulderstand on Right Bar.* Proceed as in the exercise described in the last paragraph until you come nearly to the bent arm handstand, then move a little to the right, place the right shoulder on the bar in front of the right hand, and hollow the back completely, getting almost the whole weight on the right shoulder. The shoulderstand

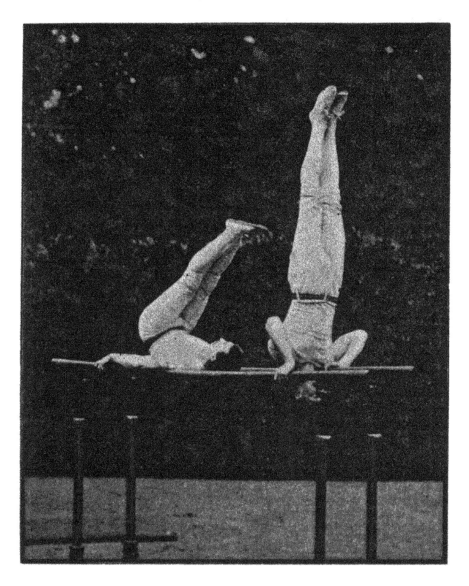

Fig. 21 —RIGHT SHOULDERSTAND AND POSITION REFERRED TO IN §§ 385, 393, 394, 498, 499, 508.

on the right bar is shown in Fig. 21. In this position the

bar should be close to the neck, so that the weight is supported on the muscle which runs from the back of the neck to the shoulder. You must get the head exactly upside down, so that you are looking straight backwards, with the head and shoulders in a completely different position from that in which they are in a handstand with bent arms.

§ 387. *From the Rest, Lift to Bent Arm Handstand.* From the rest, bend at the waist, raise the hips, and come to the bent arm handstand. This movement is just like that described in § 385, except that the legs are together all the time, which makes it a trifle more difficult. A similar lift may, of course, be done to a shoulderstand or double shoulderstand.

§ 388. *From the Riding Rest, Hands in Front, Hollow Back Lift to Bent Arm Handstand.* From the riding rest, gradually raise the body and legs to the bent arm handstand, keeping the back hollow all the time, and closing the legs gradually as you rise. A similar movement may, of course, be done to a shoulderstand or double shoulderstand.

§ 389. *From the Rest, Hollow Back Lift to Bent Arm Handstand.* From the rest, raise the body and legs to the bent arm handstand, keeping the back hollow all the way. You pass, of course, through a front lever in the rest. You may do a similar lift to a shoulderstand or double shoulderstand.

§ 390. You may do the exercises described in §§ 385, 387–389 to a handstand with straight arms. You should try to bend the arms as little as you can as you do the movement, but it is very seldom that any of these movements are accomplished with straight arms all the way. The handstand with straight arms is shown in Fig. 22. I may point out that the expression "handstand," used alone, means a handstand with straight arms.

§ 391. You may do the movements described in §§ 387, 389 from a bent arm rest, and may even lift to a handstand

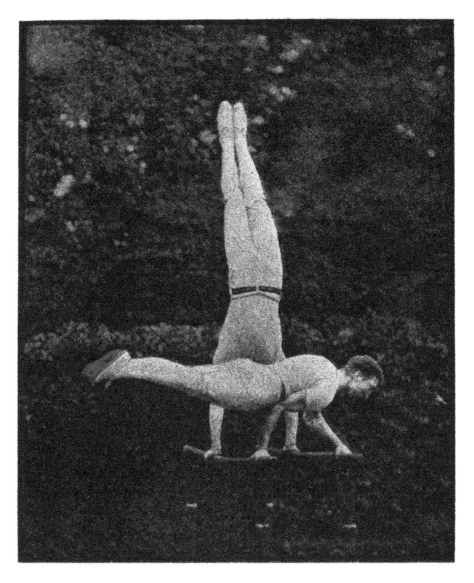

Fig. 22.—HANDSTAND AND RIGHT ELBOW LEVER.

with straight arms from the bent arm rest, either with or without a hollow back, straightening the arms gradually as you lift.

§ 392. You may return from a handstand or shoulder-stand to a rest or riding rest, with or without a hollow back, and you may stop on the way in a front lever in the rest. You may also lift from a front lever in the rest to a hand-stand or a shoulderstand.

§ 393. *From the Double Shoulderstand, Slow Roll over Forwards.* Come to the double shoulderstand, then over-balance forward and bring the hands in front of the shoulders, as described in § 385, and remain in the second position shown in Fig. 21. You may then continue as you please. This movement is a little difficult, because you must be very accurately balanced while you shift the hands, or you will not be able to retain the last-mentioned position.

§ 394. *From the Upper Arm Rest, Slow Roll Over Backwards to Double Shoulderstand.* From the upper arm rest, raise the feet to the second position shown in Fig. 21, then overbalance slightly backwards, let go with the hands, roll over on the upper arms and place the hands behind the shoulders, at the same time hollowing the back, coming to the double shoulderstand. This exercise is merely the reverse of that described in the last paragraph ; as in that exercise, you must be careful to keep the elbows well out while you shift the hands.

§ 395. *From the Shoulderstand on Right Bar, Roll over to Riding Seat on Right Bar.* Come to the shoulderstand mentioned, then bend at the waist, turn the head up so as to look at the toes, and slowly roll over until you lie along the bar, then let the legs drop one on each side of the bar, let go with the hands and rise to the riding seat on the right bar, placing the left hand on the left bar opposite the hips to steady yourself as you rise to the seat.

§ 396. You may, with a movement similar to that

described in the last paragraph, come to a cross seat instead of a riding seat, or you may drop off to the ground. Again, when the back has come in contact with the bar you may return the way you came, and arrive again in the shoulder-stand. A similar movement may also be done, with a hollow back all the way, and you may, after this movement, return with a hollow back to the shoulderstand.

§ 397. *From Upper Arm Rest, with Hands Behind, Raise Legs to Double Shoulderstand, with Arms in Upper Arm Rest, with Hands Behind.* From the upper arm rest mentioned, raise the body and legs until they are straight above your head; this you may do with a hollow back, or bending at the waist. With a hollow back it is extremely difficult. The position you reach is very like an ordinary double shoulderstand, but the arms are nearly straight, and the hands do not grasp the bar. From this position you may bend the arms, grasp the bars, and come to the ordinary double shoulderstand, or you may do a slow roll over forwards, in a manner similar to that described in § 393.

EXERCISES IN HANDSTAND AND SHOULDERSTAND.

§ 398. *From Bent Arm Handstand, Lift to Handstand with Straight Arms.* Come to the handstand with bent arms and then straighten the arms. You may, of course, also sink from a handstand with straight arms to a hand-stand with bent arms.

§ 399. In a handstand with straight or bent arms, you may travel along the bar, either walking (that is, shifting one hand at a time) or jumping (that is, shifting both hands at once). The travels forwards are much the easiest. In the bent arm handstand the jumping travel is not much more difficult than the walk, but in the straight arm hand-stand the jump is very difficult.

§ 400. *In the Bent .Arm Handstand, Travel with Alternate Shoulderstands on Right and Left Bars.* Come to a shoulderstand on the right bar, then shift the left hand either forwards or backwards, and lift the weight over to a shoulderstand on the left bar, then shift the right hand, and so on.

§ 401. From the handstand with straight arms you may turn to a handstand on one bar, or *vice versâ*, and in this way you may turn right round in the handstand. These movements are difficult. It is useful in a gymnasium to have a pair of parallel bars about 6 in. high on which to learn these movements.

§ 402. In the shoulderstand on one bar, you may let go with either hand and retain the shoulderstand.

§ 403. *From the Shoulderstand on Right Bar, Turn to Stand on the Back of the Neck on Off Bar with Hands on Near Bar.* From the shoulderstand on the right bar turn slightly to the left (that is, pass the left shoulder somewhat forwards), at the same time bend slightly at the waist, then let go with the right hand, turn further and place the right hand on the left bar close to the left hand and shift the left hand a little forward, you are then supported on the back of the neck on the off bar with the head between the bars.

§ 404. From the stand on the back of the neck on the off bar with the hands on the near bar, you may turn to the shoulderstand; this is merely the reverse of the exercise described in the last paragraph. You may, by combining this exercise with that described in the last paragraph, turn right round from the shoulderstand on the right shoulder to a shoulderstand on the same bar on the left shoulder. Again, from the stand on the back of the neck mentioned, you may let the body and legs sink till you reach a horizontal position with the back towards the ground, from which you may either let go and drop to the ground or return again to the stand on the neck. Sinking in this manner to a horizontal position puts great strain on the bars, and should, therefore, only be attempted on a thoroughly strong pair.

§ 405. *From the Shoulderstand on Right Bar, Shift to Shoulderstand on Right Shoulder on Left Bar.* From the shoulderstand on the right bar, come to the bent arm handstand, lift the head over the left bar in front of the left hand, and place the right shoulder on the left bar in front of the left hand.

§ 406. *From the Shoulderstand on Right Shoulder on Left Bar, Turn to Stand on Chest on Off Bar with Hands on Near Bar.* From the shoulderstand on the right shoulder on the left bar, turn slightly to the right (that is, move the left shoulder slightly backwards), and, at the same time shift the right hand slightly forwards, then turn further, let go with the left hand, and place it on the right bar ; you are then supported on the upper part of the chest on one bar, with the head outside the bars, and the hands on the other bar.

§ 407. From the stand on the chest on the off bar with the hands on the near bar you may turn to a shoulderstand on the right shoulder on the left bar ; this is merely the reverse of the last exercise. By means of this exercise, and that described in the last paragraph, you may turn right round. From the same stand on the chest, you may let the body and legs sink till you reach a horizontal position with the back towards the ground ; this exercise requires exceptional strength, and puts an immense strain on the bars.

§ 408. You may reach the stand on the chest, described

m § 406, from a front rest on the near bar with reverse grasp, by letting the shoulders fall forward, till the top of the chest rests against the off bar, and then raising the body and legs. From the same stand on the chest you may let go, at the same time bending the waist, and drop in front of the off bar, catching it with the hands as you drop, so that you come to a hang on the off bar with reverse grasp, and with the legs in half lever.

§ 409. *From the Back Rest on Off Bar, Fall Back, and Raise Feet to Stand on Neck on Near Bar with Hands on Off Bar.* From the back rest on the off bar, let the shoulders fall back, and come in contact with the near bar, then raise the legs above the head, with the back as nearly hollow as possible. From this position you may bend at the waist, and let the feet pass to the outside of the near bar, and then let go, and drop on the feet outside the near bar.

ELBOW LEVERS.

§ 410. *From the Riding Rest, Hands in Front, Rise to Double Elbow Lever.* From the rest mentioned, raise the legs nearly as if you intended to do a front lever in the rest, but, as you raise the legs, close the elbows somewhat, so that you support yourself in a horizontal position on your elbows.

§ 411. *From the Outside Rest Behind Right Hand, Rise to Right Elbow Lever.* Come to the position named, then do a quarter left turn, slightly bending the right elbow, and bringing it as far to the left under the body as you can, then lean slightly forward, and raise the feet until you reach a horizontal position with the back hollow. The right elbow lever is shown in Fig. 22 ; it is a difficult position to reach at first. In the position you must keep the head well up, and, if anything, higher than the feet; and you must keep the whole body and the legs quite at right angles to the bars. The tendency at first is to get the head too low and too far to the right. In reaching the elbow lever, in the manner described above, you must turn as you begin the movement, and take care never to get the head lower than its ultimate position. You will not at first be able to tell for yourself whether you are really horizontal in an elbow lever.

§ 412. You may in the right elbow lever let go with the left hand altogether, and do the lever entirely on the right arm. The position you then reach is called a "free right elbow lever." In this position the left arm should be held out in a straight line with the body and legs.

§ 413. *From the Riding Rest, Hands in Front, Rise to Right Elbow Lever.* From the riding rest mentioned, turn to the left, bringing the right elbow under the stomach, then raise the legs, and turn further to the left, closing the legs, and hollowing the back, coming to the elbow lever.

§ 414. From the right elbow lever you may lift to a handstand or shoulderstand; the only point requiring mention about these movements is that the back must be kept hollow the whole time. You may also sink to an elbow lever from the shoulderstand or handstand.

§ 415. From the right elbow lever you may carry the feet to the rear, still supporting the weight on the elbow until the body is parallel to the bars, and then shift the weight slightly to the left, coming to a double elbow lever, or to a front lever in the rest.

§ 416. You may pass from the right elbow lever to the left elbow lever. This is merely a continuation of the last exercise; at first you will find it exceedingly difficult to manage without getting the feet considerably higher than the head as you pass from the one elbow to the other; but this you should try to avoid. The body should be horizontal throughout the movement.

§ 417. From the free right elbow lever you may bring the left hand on to the right bar, and shift the weight on to the left elbow, passing through a double elbow lever on the right bar, and so reach the left elbow lever on the bar which was originally the right bar. In this manner you may, of course, turn completely round.

§ 418. From the free right elbow lever you may let the feet pass to the rear, pivoting about the right arm until the body is parallel to the bar, then take hold of the right bar with the left hand, and lift to a handstand on the right bar alone, continuing with an overthrow, or squat, or other movements.

§ 419. From the free right elbow lever you may place the left hand on the right bar behind the right hand, and then rise to a shoulderstand on the right bar, grasping the right bar with combined grasp throughout the movement.

§ 420. You may rise from a side seat on the right bar to a free right elbow lever without using the left hand at all; this movement is, however, extremely difficult.

PART III.—*QUICK EXERCISES.*

§§ 421–428. Vaults from Rest to Ground—§§ 429–451. Leg Circles, etc., in Cross Positions—§§ 452–474. Vaults, Leg Circles, etc., from Side Positions—§§ 475–481. Vaults and Leg Circles with Turns—§§ 482–492. Swinging Exercises from Rest—493–497. Exercises between Rest and Hang—§§ 498–515. Upper

Arm Swings, etc.—§§ 516–521. Swinging Exercises with Turns—§§ 522–531. Miscellaneous Exercises— § 532. Combined Exercises.

VAULTS FROM REST TO GROUND.

§ 421. *From the Rest, Swing, and Rear Vault in Front of Right Hand.* From the rest, take a slight swing, and carry the legs over the right bar in front of the right hand with the legs horizontal and the back of the legs towards the bar, let go with both hands, hollow the back sharply, place the left hand on the right bar, and alight. The vault is just like a rear vault over the horizontal bar.

§ 422. *From the Rest, Swing, and Rear Vault in Front of Right Hand, with Quarter, Half, or Complete Left Turn.* Begin as in the last exercise; when you let go with both hands, however, turn sharply to the left. If you do a quarter turn, grasp the right bar with both hands as you alight; if you do a half left turn, grasp it with the right hand; if you do a complete turn, grasp it with the left hand. In these exercises you should endeavour to hollow the back the moment you let go, and to finish your turn completely before you alight. A left turn after a rear vault in front of the right hand is often called an "inside turn." The rear vault with a complete inside turn is extremely difficult.

§ 423. *From the Rest, Swing, and Flank Vault in Front of Right Hand.* From the rest, take a moderate swing; when the legs have nearly reached the forward extremity of their swing, let go with the left hand, and do a quarter right turn very sharply, at the same time hollowing the back, then carry the body over the right bar, and alight. From the moment you have done your quarter right turn, the movement is exactly like a flank vault over the horizontal bar; you alight clear of the bars with your back towards them.

§ 424. *From the Rest, Swing, and Front Vault in Front of Right Hand.* From the rest, take a good swing, when the legs have nearly reached the forward extremity of their swing, let go with the left hand, and do a half right turn, at the same time hollowing the back very sharply, then carry the body over the right bar, and alight. From the moment you have done your half right turn, the movement is exactly like a front vault over the horizontal bar. This is an extremely pretty vault if well done, but it is not at all easy. You must keep the weight well over the right arm, so that you are for an instant carried on the right arm over the right bar in a horizontal position with the back hollow, and the face towards the ground. As you turn you must shift the grasp of the right hand, so that, as you descend, the back of the hand is towards the other bar. Beginners in attempting this vault generally do almost a complete rear vault, and then do a half right turn; and this movement looks extremely clumsy.

§ 425. *From the Rest, Swing, and Front Vault in Front of Right Hand with Half Right Turn.* Begin as in the last exercise, but, as you make your half right turn, let go with both hands, and do another half right turn as you descend, grasp the bar with the left hand, and alight. The back should be hollow throughout the exercise from the moment you let go. This turn is often called an "outside turn."

§ 426. *From the Rest, Swing and Front Vault behind Right Hand.* From the rest, take a swing and carry the legs over the right bar behind the right hand; as the legs pass over the bar push sharply from the hands and let go, place the left hand on the right bar, and alight. The main difficulty about the movement is to keep the back perfectly hollow while descending. You should alight just opposite the place where your hands were originally.

§ 427. *From the Rest, Swing and Front Vault behind Right Hand with a Half Left Turn.* Proceed as in the exercise described in the last paragraph, but do not let go with the right hand, and, as soon as you have let go with the left hand, do a half turn sharply, and alight, still holding with the right hand. The movement, which is easy, is like the screw vault over the horizontal bar, described in § 243. This turn is often called an " outside turn."

§ 428. *From the Rest, Swing and Front Vault behind Right Hand with Half Right Turn.* Begin as in the exercise described in § 426, then, the moment you let go with both hands, do a half right turn sharply, take hold of the right bar with the right hand, and alight. This turn is often called an " inside turn."

LEG CIRCLES, ETC., IN CROSS POSITIONS.

§ 429. Leg circles may be done on the parallel bars similar in character to leg circles on the horse or horizontal bar. The variety of these movements is very great, and it is accordingly necessary to adopt a somewhat artificial system of nomenclature in describing them. The general explanation of this system I shall postpone till § 443, where it will be more conveniently discussed ; in the mean time I shall discuss one series of leg circles, in the description of which there is little difficulty.

§ 430. *From the Cross Stand at Near End of Bars, Forward Leg Circle over Left Bar to Half Lever.*

(i.) *With Left Leg.* From the cross stand mentioned, spring, separate the legs, carry the left leg forward outside the left bar, raising the left hand to let it pass, and at the same time carry the right leg forward between the bars, let the legs meet in the half lever, and remain there. Through-out the movement the two legs should move together, so that at any moment a straight line joining the feet would be horizontal, and at right angles to the bars.

(ii.) *With Right Leg in Front of Left Leg.* From the cross stand mentioned, spring, carry the right leg in front of the left outside the left bar, raising the left hand to let it pass, and, at the same time, carry the left leg forward between the bars; when the right leg is clear of the bar the legs will be crossed with the right leg over the left, both legs being nearly horizontal, then uncross the legs and remain in the half lever.

(iii.) *With Right Leg Behind Left Leg.* From the cross stand mentioned, spring, carry the right leg behind the left leg outside the left bar, raising the left hand to let it pass, and, at the same time, carry the left leg forward between the bars; when the right leg is clear of the bar the legs will be crossed with the right leg under the left, then uncross the legs and remain in the half lever. This is rather a difficult movement; you must raise the hips rather high when you spring, so that, while the right leg is passing outside the left bar, the bar is between the calves of the legs.

(iv.) *With Both Legs.* From the cross stand mentioned, spring, carry both legs outside the left bar, raising the left hand to let them pass, and remain in the half lever.

§ 431. *From Cross Stand at Near End of Bars, Straddle Forwards to Half Lever.* From the cross stand mentioned, spring, straddle the legs, and carry them forward outside the bars, the right leg passing outside the right bar and the left outside the left bar, replace the hands, and let the legs meet in a half lever, and remain there. This exercise is like that on the horse, described in § 111.

§ 432. The exercises described in the last two paragraphs

need not lead to the half lever. In the first place, as will appear in § 442, you need not replace the left hand at all, in which case you do not even reach a momentary half lever, properly so called. Secondly, you may reach a momentary half lever and continue without pausing in it. However, it is most important to learn to remain in the half lever after these movements, because, if you can so remain, you will find that you have acquired such control over the movements that you will be able to bring them into combination with other movements with the greatest ease. In beginning these movements you should stand perfectly upright just so far from the end of the bars that you can take hold of the bars with the arms almost, but not absolutely, straight, then bend the knees slightly, and spring. Do not get into the habit of taking preliminary jumps, or of running at the bars, or of taking your position with the body bent at the waist. When you reach the half lever you should remain there absolutely stationary.

§ 433. Movements similar to those described in §§ 430, 431, may be done from a rest at the near end of the bars. For these exercises you must take a very slight swing, at the same time raising the hips slightly, so that the preparatory movement is rather a movement of the hips to the rear than a real swing.

§ 434. Movements similar to those described in the last paragraph may be done from the rest at the centre of the bars. From this position forward circles with both legs or with the right leg over the left bar are difficult, as is also the straddle forwards. You want, of course, rather more swing than for the same movements at the near end of the bars, but you must take as little swing as possible.

§ 435. The circles described in the last paragraph may also be done from a rest with one leg or both legs over the right bar behind the right hand; that is, from the rests numbered vii., x., xiii., and xiv. in § 363. They may also be done from a front leaning rest.

§ 436. Forward circles over one bar and the straddle forwards may also be done at the further end of the bars, either to a half lever or momentary half lever, or to the ground, with or without a turn. In doing forward circles over the left bar to the ground without a turn take a moderate swing, and, the moment you are clear of the left bar, let go with the right hand, hollow the back sharply, and alight with your back to the bars; you do not, of course, replace the left hand. In doing·these movements with a quarter right turn you should retain the grasp with the right hand, and in doing these movements with a quarter left turn you should replace the left hand and let go with the right hand. In doing a forward straddle to the ground, you should take a moderate swing, and, the moment you raise the hands, hollow the back very sharply, and close the legs in the air, so that you assume a vertical position before you alight.

§ 437. *From the Half Lever at Near End of Bars, Backward Circles over Left Bar to Ground.* You may do movements of this kind with the left leg, with the right leg in front of the left leg, with the right leg behind the left leg, or with both legs. These movements are easy, they are simply the reverse of the movements described in § 430. You must lean well back as you begin, and get the weight well on the right hand, take hold of the left bar again as you descend, and be careful that you alight upright with both feet together, and with the shoulders at right angles to the bars. You may do similar movements without replacing the left hand, with a quarter left turn as you alight.

§ 438. *From the Half Lever at Near End of Bars,*

Straddle Backwards to Ground. From the position mentioned, lean well back, straddle the legs and carry them backwards, the right leg outside the right bar, and the left outside the left bar, letting go with both hands, and alight. This is simply the reverse of the exercise described in § 431. It is very easy, but a little dangerous at first.

§ 439. Exercises similar to those described in the last two paragraphs may be done to the rest instead of to the ground. You must make your movement quickly, and must, of course, not lean back. It is by no means easy to do a backward circle with both legs, or the straddle backwards to the rest, without touching the bars with the legs.

§ 440. Exercises similar to those described in the last paragraph may be done at the centre of the bars or at the further end, but they are extremely difficult to do without touching the bars with the legs. Indeed, I have never seen any of them done clear, except the backward circle with the left leg over the left bar, and, of course, the corresponding exercise right. However, although there is generally a graze in doing the exercises, they are sometimes very neat and effective.

§ 441. The exercises described in §§ 430–440 may be combined in various ways.

(i.) Forward circles over the left bar may be followed by forward circles over the same bar, or over the other bar, letting the legs swing back from the half lever between each circle. These exercises may be done at the centre of the bars, or at either end.

(ii.) At the near end of the bars, forward circles may be followed by backward circles to the ground over the same bar, or over the other bar, without pause in the half lever.

(iii.) Backward circles over one bar may be followed by

forward circles over the other bar. These exercises may be done at the centre of the bars, or at either end.

(iv.) Backward circles with the right leg over the left bar may be followed by a forward circle with the left leg over the left bar.

(v.) A forward straddle may be followed by forward circles over either bar, or by another forward straddle, letting the legs swing back from the half lever between the movements. These exercises may be done at the centre, or at either end of the bars.

(vi.) Forward circles may be followed by a forward straddle, letting the legs swing back between the movements. These exercises may be done at the centre, or at either end of the bars, but, except at the further end of the bars, are very difficult.

(vii.) At the near end of the bars, forward circles may be followed by a back straddle to the ground. These combinations are not very difficult, and are effective. There should be no perceptible pause in the half lever.

(viii.) Forward circles may be followed by a backward straddle to the rest. These combinations are very difficult. They are possible at the centre, or at either end of the bars, but the straddle backwards is, as I have said, almost impossible to do clear, except at the near end of the bars.

(ix.) At the near end of the bars, a forward straddle may be followed by a backward straddle to the ground. This is a very pretty but difficult movement. There should be no pause in the half lever.

(x.) A forward straddle might be followed by a backward straddle to the rest, but I do not think I have ever seen this movement done clear, even at the near end of the bars.

(xi.) A backward straddle to the rest might be followed

by forward circles or by a forward straddle, but I do not
think I have ever seen these combinations done.

§ 442. Forward circles over the left bar may be combined with vaults over the right bar in front of the right
hand, without replacing the left hand on the left bar. These
exercises may be done from the ground at the near end
of the bars ; or from the rest, either at the near end, or
the centre, of the bars. Where a forward circle with both
legs over the one bar is immediately followed by a vault
over the other, in the manner described above, the whole
movement is called a vault over both bars for shortness'
sake ; for example, a forward circle with both legs over the
left bar, followed, without replacing the left hand on the left
bar, by a rear vault to ground in front of the right hand, is
called "rear vault over both bars to ground in front of
right hand." These movements are easiest at the near end
of the bars from the ground, most difficult at the centre of
the bars. They are easiest with a rear vault, and most
difficult with a front vault. Vaults over both bars at the
centre of the bars are not very difficult to accomplish, but
are extremely difficult to do well ; indeed, I have hardly
ever seen these movements done to perfection even by
the finest gymnasts. The great difficulties are to keep the
legs straight and closed, especially at the beginning of the
movement, to avoid getting the hips too high, and to keep
the head up. All the movements described in this paragraph resemble double rear vaults and other similar movements on the horse.

§ 443. In the present paragraph I shall explain the
general system upon which all leg circles on the parallel
bars may be described. All leg circles on the parallel bars
may be called right or left, according as the circling is with
the hands of a watch, or against the hands of a watch.

P

Now these movements are so numerous and varied that it is necessary to lay down the following rules with regard to them—

(i.) In right or left circles with one leg the other leg, in the absence of directions to the contrary, remains in its original position, as nearly as may be, throughout the movement.

(ii.) If the circle is said to be "over one bar," the circling leg or legs must not pass over the other bar. For example, in a right circle over the right bar from a cross position you must carry the circling leg or legs forwards between the bars, and backwards outside the right bar; again, in a right circle over the near bar from a side position you must carry the circling leg or legs to the right between the bars, and to the left outside the near bar.

(iii.) If the circle is said to be "over both bars," the circling leg or legs must not move in the direction of the bars between the bars. For example, in a right circle over both bars from a cross position you must carry the circling leg or legs forwards outside the left bar, and backwards outside the right bar.

(iv.) You may, of course, do complete right or left circles over one bar or both bars, returning to the position from which you started, and if you are told to do such and such a circle, without words to indicate where the movement is to conclude, you are intended to do a complete circle. On the other hand, you may do a portion of a complete circle only, and such a movement is generally described as a "circle right" or "circle left," to the position you are intended to reach. However, in some cases, the portion of a complete circle may be sufficiently described without stating the concluding position; in the first place, if the circle is said to be "over right and left bars," or "over left and right bars," you must proceed as in a circle over both bars, until you have brought the circling leg or legs between the bars after passing the last mentioned bar, when the movement is considered to be complete; secondly, in descriptions of some exercises the expression "half circle" is employed, as will appear later. The diagram (Fig. 23) will serve to explain this paragraph more clearly. This diagram shows a plan of the parallel bars. The one dotted line shows a plan of a circle over the one bar, the other dotted line the plan of a circle over the other bar, and the solid line a plan of a circle over both bars. In a circle "over the left and right bars" the movement is complete as soon as you have brought the

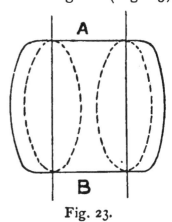

Fig. 23.

circling leg or legs either to the point A or to the point B.

§ 444. It is obvious that the forward and backward circles, described in §§ 430–440, might be described upon the system explained in the last paragraph, but the description would be extremely cumbrous, because it would be necessary, in the case of such circles with one leg, to mention the movement of the other leg, and also, as a rule, to mention the concluding position.

§ 445. A variety of leg circles may be done from rests with one leg or both legs over the right bar, either in front of or behind the right hand. In the next few paragraphs I shall give examples of these movements.

§ 446. *From the Outside Rest in Front of Right Hand.*

(i.) *Left Circle with Left Leg over Right Bar.* From the rest mentioned (vi. in § 363), pass the left leg over the right bar to the left, swing it back between the bars, pass it over the right bar behind the right hand, continue the swing of the left leg, raising the right hand and right leg for a moment to let the leg pass underneath, and return to your original position. This is a very difficult movement.

(ii.) *Right Circle with Left Leg over Right Bar.* From the rest mentioned, raise the legs and right hand for a moment from the bar, pass the left leg back underneath the right, replace the right hand and leg, pass the left leg over the right bar, swing it forwards between the bars, and pass it over the right bar again, returning to your original position. This is also difficult.

(iii.) *Left Circle with Right Leg over Right Bar.* From the rest mentioned, raise both legs, pass the right leg under the left leg and over the right bar, swing it back between the bars and over the right bar behind the right hand, raise the right hand for an instant to let the leg pass, and return to your original position.

(iv.) *Right Circle with Right Leg over Right Bar.* From the rest mentioned, pass the right leg backwards, raising the right hand to let it pass, pass it over the right bar behind the right hand, swing it forwards between the bars, and pass it over the right bar again to the original position, raising the left leg to let it pass.

§ 447. *From the Outside Rest Behind Right Hand.*

(i.) *Right Circle with Left Leg over Right Bar.* It is sufficiently obvious how to do this.

(ii.) *Right Circle with Left Leg over Both Bars.* Pass the left leg under the right leg and over both bars behind you, then forwards outside the left bar, raising the left hand, then over both bars in front of you, and backwards outside the right bar, raising the right hand to let it pass, and return to your original position.

(iii.) *Left Circle with Left Leg over Right Bar.* This movement is obvious.

(iv.) *Left Circle with Left Leg over Both Bars.* This movement is obvious.

§ 448. From the rest with the legs in riding seat on right bar in front of or behind right hand, circles can be done with either leg over the right bar. Further, right and left circles can be done with the left leg over the left bar, or over both bars. These movements hardly want full description. In circles over the left bar, the circling leg passes forwards outside the left bar and backwards between bars, or *vice versâ*. In circles over both bars, the circling leg passes forwards outside the left bar and backwards outside the right bar, or *vice versâ*.

§ 449. Circles similar to those described in the last paragraph can be done from other rests with one leg over one bar.

§ 450. From the riding seat with the hands behind or in front, you may do circles over one bar or both bars with one leg.

§ 451. The exercises described in §§ 446–450 may be combined with forward and backward circles and vaults. The following are examples of such combinations—

(i.) From the Rest at Centre of Bars, Swing, Backward Circle with Left Leg over Right Bar, Forward Circle with Left Leg over Left Bar (this brings you to a momentary half lever), Swing Back, Circle with Left Leg over Both Bars Right to Rest with Left Leg over Right Bar in Front of Right Hand, Circle with Right Leg over Right Bar Left to Rest with Legs Astride Right Arm, Circle with Left Leg over Right Bar Left to Outside Rest behind Right Hand, and Rear Vault over Both Bars to Ground in Front of Right Hand.

(ii.) From Cross Stand at Near End of Bars, Straddle Forwards, Swing Back, Circle with Both Legs over Left

Bar Right to Outside of Left Bar, and Circle with Right
Leg over Both Bars Right to Riding Seat with Right Hand
behind Right Leg (this is the first time either leg touches
the bar), Place Hands in Front of Legs, Right Circle with
Right Leg over Right and Left Bars, Circle with Right Leg
over Left Bar Right to join Left Leg, Circle with Both Legs
over Left Bar Right to Momentary Half Lever, Swing
Back, and Flank Vault over Both Bars to Ground in Front
of Right Hand (the right leg does not touch the bars after
it is raised from the right bar).

VAULTS, LEG CIRCLES, ETC., FROM SIDE POSITIONS.

§ 452. *Vaults, etc., over Near Bar with Hands on Near
Bar.* From the side stand at the side of the bars with
hands on the near bar, or from the front rest on the near
bar, you may do a flank vault, or squat or straddle, over the
near bar to a side stand between the bars. In the left flank
vault you should shift the left hand on to the off bar as
soon as you raise it from the near bar, so as to guide the
body while descending, and then shift the right hand on to
the off bar just before you alight. In the squat or straddle,
you should shift both hands on to the off bar as soon as
you let go the near bar. Similar movements may be done
to a rest on the off bar.

§ 453. *Vaults, etc., over Both Bars with Hands on Near
Bar.* From the side stand at the side of the bars with the
hands on the near bar, you may do flank, front, or rear
vaults, or squat or straddle, over both bars to the ground.
These exercises are most easily done with a run.

§ 454. *Leg Circles, etc., over Both Bars with Hands on
Near Bar.* From the side stand at the side of the bars
with the hands on the near bar, or from the rest on the

near bar, you may do a half circle with both legs, or squat over both bars to a back rest on the near bar with the legs over the off bar. You may do similar exercises, letting go the near bar in the course of the movement, and coming to a side seat or back rest on the off bar. You may also, from the same positions, straddle over both bars to a side seat on the off bar, but, after this movement, you alight very heavily on the off bar, and you should therefore only attempt it on a very strong pair of bars.

§ 455. *Springs to Rest on Off Bar with Legs over Near Bar.* From the side stand at the side of the bars with the hands on the near bar, you may spring to the rest on the off bar with the legs over the near bar. This is an easy movement, but requires some little practice to enable you to reach a position from which you can continue without pause with the movements hereafter to be described. Again, from the side stand at the side of the bars, without touching the bars, you may spring, place the hands on the off bar, and reach the rest on the off bar with the legs over the near bar. This exercise is most easily done with a run.

§ 456. *Vaults, etc., over Near Bar from Rest on Off Bar with Legs over Near Bar.* From the rest on the off bar with the legs over the near bar, you may do a flank vault, or squat or straddle over the near bar to a side stand between the bars, or to the rest on the off bar. In doing these movements you must spring from the thighs and carry the legs over the near bar; in squatting or straddling in this manner, you must raise the hips rather high.

§ 457. *Vaults, etc., over Both Bars from Rest on Off Bar with Legs over Near Bar.* From the rest on the off bar with the legs over the near bar you may do flank, rear, front, or screw vaults, or squat or straddle, over both bars to the ground. These are not very difficult movements. You must get the weight well forward, spring from the thighs, and carry the legs over both bars, alighting outside the off bar. From the same position, you may do a circle with both legs over both bars, right or left, or squat or straddle over both bars, to a back rest on the off bar.

§ 458. The exercises described in the last two paragraphs may be combined with those described in § 455, with no perceptible pause in the rest. These movements are very pretty, and not very difficult.

§ 459. *Vaults, etc., over Near Bar from Side Stand outside Bars with Hands on Off Bar.* From a side stand at the side of the bars you may spring, place the hands on the off bar, and do a flank vault, or squat, or straddle over the near bar to the side stand between the bars, or to the rest on the off bar, without letting the legs touch the near bar. These movements are most easily done with a run.

§ 460. *Vaults, etc., over Both Bars from Side Stand outside Bars with Hands on Off Bar.* From the side stand outside the bars, you may spring, place the hands on the off bar, and do flank, front, rear, or screw vaults, or squat or straddle, over both bars to the ground. These exercises are most easily done with a run ; they do not, of course, lend themselves to combination with other exercises, but they are effective movements. You may also, in a similar manner, do a circle over both bars with both legs, or squat or straddle, to a back rest on the off bar.

§ 461. *From the Rest on Off Bar with Legs over Near Bar.*

(i.) *Right Circle with Left Leg over Near Bar.* Carry the left leg over the near bar to the left, swing it to the right between the bars, and carry it over the near bar again to the right, raise the right leg to let it pass, and return to your original position.

(ii.) *Left Circle with Left Leg over Near Bar.* This is a similar movement to that last described. The left leg begins by passing under the right.

Half of either of these circles will bring you from the rest mentioned to a rest on the off bar with one leg over the near bar, and such a movement may be conveniently described as a " half circle."

§ 462. *Leg Circles over Near Bar from Rest on Off Bar with One Leg over Near Bar.* You may do circles with the left leg from the rest on the off bar with the right leg over the near bar; these are practically the same movements as those described in the last paragraph. Half of one of these movements will bring you from the rest mentioned to a rest on the off bar with the legs over the near bar, and such a movement may be conveniently described as a half circle. Again, from the same position, you may carry the right leg over the near bar either to the right or to the left, coming to a side stand between the bars or to the rest on the off bar. Such a movement may also be conveniently described as a half circle.

§ 463. *Vaults, etc., over Both Bars from Rest on Off Bar with One Leg over Near Bar.* From the rest on the off bar with the right leg over near bar, you may do flank, front, rear, or screw vaults over both bars to the ground, either left or right. You must swing the left leg, which is between the bars, a little to get the start, then carry the left leg over the off bar and the right leg over both bars, alighting outside the off bar, closing the legs as you pass over the off bar. These movements are not difficult. From the same position you may, in a similar manner, circle the left leg over the off bar and the right leg over both bars simultaneously to a back rest on the off bar.

§ 464. The circles and half circles described in §§ 461,

462, may be combined with the vaults described in §§ 456, 457, and 463, without pause, for example—

(i.) From the Rest on Off Bar with Legs over Near Bar, Right Circle over Near Bar with Right Leg, and Flank Vault Left over Both Bars to Ground. This is an easy exercise.

(ii.) From Rest on Off Bar with Legs over Near Bar, Left Circle over Near Bar with Right Leg, and Flank Vault Right over Near Bar to Side Stand between Bars. This is very difficult to do without letting either leg touch the near bar after the left leg is raised to let the right leg pass.

(iii.) From Rest on Off Bar with Legs over Near Bar, Half Right Circle over Near Bar with Right Leg, and Rear Vault Right over Both Bars to Ground.

§ 465. *Vaults, etc., over Off Bar from Side Stand between Bars, and from Rest on Off Bar.* From the side stand between bars with hands on off bar, or from the rest on the off bar, you may do vaults, or leg circles, or squat or straddle, over the off bar. These movements are just like similar movements on a horizontal bar, but the bar behind your back is a little baulking at first.

§ 466. *From the Side Stand between Bars with Hands on Off Bar.*

(i.) *Half Right Circle with Right Leg over Near Bar to Rest on Off Bar with Right Leg over Near Bar.* Spring, and carry the right leg to the right and over the near bar backwards, coming to the position indicated.

(ii.) *Half Left Circle with Right Leg over Near Bar to Rest on Off Bar with Right Leg over Near Bar.* Spring, and carry the right leg to the left behind the left and over the near bar backwards to the position indicated.

(iii.) *Half Right Circle with Both Legs to Rest on Off Bar with Legs over Near Bar.* This requires no further explanation.

(iv.) *Squat Back to Rest on Off Bar with Legs over Near Bar.* You must raise the hips high and bring the feet up almost exactly as if you were going to do a squat over the off bar, but when the feet come as high as the bar shoot them sharply out backwards.

(v.) *Straddle Back to Rest on Off Bar with Legs over Near Bar.* Spring and instantly straddle the legs, and carry them over the near bar backwards, close them, and let them come in contact with the near bar.

§ 467. The exercises (iii.), (iv.), and (v.), described in the last paragraph, may, of course, be done to the ground on the outside of the near bar, and, in alighting, you may make various turns.

§ 468. *From the Side Stand between Bars with Hands on Off Bar.*

(i.) *Right Circle with Right Leg over Near Bar to Ground.* Begin as in exercise (i.) in § 466, but carry the leg right round without touching the bar, and come to the ground again in your original position.

(ii.) *Left Circle with Right Leg over Near Bar to Ground.* This is similar to the last exercise.

(iii.) *Left Circle with Both Legs over Near Bar to Ground.* This exercise is similar to the two last described.

§ 469. You may do the exercises described in the last paragraph, but, instead of returning to the ground, vault over the off bar; of course you do not quite complete the circle. The left circle with both legs over the near bar, followed by a right vault over the off bar, is a very pretty movement if well done. You must endeavour to show the free front lever distinctly in the course of the movement; that is to say, you must try, when your legs are straight behind you, to be perfectly horizontal, and to have the back quite hollow, just as in the free front lever on the horse, described in § 117.

§ 470. *From the Side Stand Between the Bars with Hands on Off Bar.*

(i.) *Squat Back to Free Front Lever, and Squat Forward over Near Bar to Ground.* Begin as in exercise (iv.) in § 466, but, instead of letting the legs touch the near bar, just reach the free front lever, and then return the legs over the bar and reach your original position.

(ii.) *Squat Back to Free Front Lever and Straddle Forward over Near Bar to Ground.* This is just like the last exercise, but, when you reach the free front lever, you straddle instead of squatting.

(iii.) *Straddle Back to Free Front Lever and Squat Forwards over Near Bar to Ground.*

(iv.) *Straddle Back to Free Front Lever and Straddle Forwards over Near Bar to Ground.*

§ 471. You may do the exercises described in the last paragraph, but, instead of doing the final squat or straddle over the near bar, do them over both bars and alight in front of the off bar. These are very effective movements, but are by no means easy.

§ 472. The exercises described in §§ 466–471, may be done from a rest on the off bar; but these movements are most of them extremely difficult and rather cramped.

§ 473. *Leg Circles, etc., from Back Rest on Near Bar with Legs over Off Bar.* From the position mentioned you may do leg circles, or squat or straddle backwards, over the off bar; but these movements are ineffective. From the same position you may do a circle with both legs, or squat or straddle backwards, over both bars to the ground; these movements are rather effective.

§ 474. The exercises described in §§ 452–473, lead themselves to very pretty combinations. In the first place, such of these exercises as lead to the rest on the off bar with the legs over the near bar, may be followed without pause, by the exercises which begin from that position ; in these combinations the legs should come in contact with the near bar and immediately leave it again, so that you merely strike the near bar with the legs. Secondly, such of the exercises as lead to the side stand between the bars may be followed, without pause, by the exercises which begin from that position ; in these combinations you should, of course, bend the knees slightly as you alight in the side stand between the bars ; then, as you straighten the knees again, you should spring and continue, so that you never assume a stationary position in the side stand. The following are examples of exercises of this kind—

(i.) From Side Stand at Side of Bars with Hands on Near Bar, Flank Vault Left over Near Bar to Ground and Flank Vault Right over Off Bar to Ground.

(ii.) With a Run, Spring, Place Hands on Off Bar, Flank Vault Left over Near Bar to Ground, Circle with Both Legs Right over Near Bar, and Rear Vault Left over Off Bar to Ground.

(iii.) From Side Stand at Side of Bars with Hands on Near Bar, Spring to Rest on Off Bar with Legs over Near Bar ; Straddle over Near Bar to Ground ; Straddle Back over Near Bar to Rest on Off Bar with Legs over Near Bar, and Straddle over Both Bars to Ground.

(iv.) From Side Stand at Side of Bars with Hands on Near Bar, Squat over Near Bar to Ground. Straddle Back over Near Bar to Free Front Lever ; Right Circle with Right Leg over Near Bar (letting Left Leg come in contact with Near Bar) and Front Vault Left over Both Bars to Ground.

VAULTS AND LEG CIRCLES WITH TURNS.

§ 475. *From the Side Stand outside Near Bar, Front Vault Left In.* From the side stand mentioned, take a combined grasp of the near bar with the right hand reversed, do a front vault left over the near bar, and, when you let go with the left hand, place it on the off bar ; you will then be in a momentary front lever in the rest ; if you intend to continue with a forward swing, you must try to reach the momentary front lever with the legs as high as possible, the arms straight, and the back perfectly hollow. If you wish to retain the front lever in the rest after the vault, which is very difficult, you must get the weight rather more to the right as you vault, than if you mean to continue with a swing.

§ 476. You may do the exercise described in the last paragraph, and immediately straddle the legs and come to a riding rest with hands in front, or carry one or both legs over the off bar ; these movements are described as " front vault in " to the rest ultimately reached.

§ 477. *From the Side Stand outside Near Bar, Rear Vault Right In.* Take an ordinary grasp of the near bar, and do a rear vault right over the near bar, let go with both hands at once and replace them on the bars simultaneously ; the right hand on the near bar and the left hand on the off bar, so that you reach a half lever or momentary half lever. You should learn to retain the half lever after this vault.

§ 478. You may do the exercise described in the last paragraph, and immediately straddle the legs, coming to a riding rest with hands behind, or carry one or both legs over the off bar to a rest with one leg or both legs over the left bar in front of the left hand. These movements are described as "rear vault in," to the rest ultimately reached.

§ 479. *From the Side Stand outside Near Bar, Circle with*

Both Legs over Both Bars Right with Quarter Right Turn to Half Lever. Take a combined grasp of the near bar with the right hand reversed, spring, carry the legs over the near bar to the left, letting go with the left hand; then turn the shoulders to the right and carry the legs forward outside the off bar, placing the left hand on the off bar as soon as the legs have passed over the bar.

§ 480. Many of the leg circles which have been described in former paragraphs may be combined with a turn of the body, shifting the hands as you turn. Quarter turns will of course bring you from a cross rest to a side rest, or *vice versâ*, half turns from one cross rest to another, or from one side rest to another. In all circles with one leg hitherto described, in which the other leg is outside the bars, the circling leg, if passing the other, passes between it and the bars. Now, if you do a turn as you do the circle, you may pass the circling leg outside the other, and such a leg circle is called a " screw circle." A screw circle, it should be pointed out, differs from any other circle only at the move-ment when the legs pass each other. As a rule, in describing circles with simultaneous turns, it is not necessary to say what is done with the hands, as that will generally be obvious; however, it may sometimes be necessary. The following are examples of leg circles with turns—

(i.) From Riding Rest, Hands Behind; Circle with Right Leg over Right Bar Left, with Quarter Right Turn to Front Rest on Right Bar, with Left Leg over Left Bar.

(ii.) From Riding Rest, Hands in Front; Circle with Right Leg over Both Bars Right, with Quarter Right Turn to Front Rest on Right Bar with Legs over Left Bar.

(iii.) From Rest on Off Bar with Legs over Near Bar, Circle with Left Leg over Both Bars Right, with Quarter Right Turn to Riding Rest, Hands in Front.

(iv.) From Rest on Off Bar with Legs over Near Bar, Circle with Right Leg over Both Bars Right, with Quarter Left Turn to Riding Rest, Hands Behind.

(v.) From Rest, Circle with Left Leg over Right Bar Right, with Quarter Right Turn to Side Riding Rest on Right Bar Alone.

(vi.) From Back Rest on Off Bar, Circle with Both Legs over Both Bars Right, with Quarter Right Turn to Outside Rest in Front of Right Hand.

(vii.) From Rest with Left Leg over Right Bar in Front of Right Hand, Swing Right Leg Back and Screw Circle with Right Leg over Both Bars Left with Half Left Turn, to Riding Rest, Hands in Front.

(viii.) From Rest on Off Bar with Right Leg over Near Bar, Swing Left Leg to the Left, and Screw Circle with Left Leg over Both Bars Left, with Three Quarters Left Turn to Riding Rest, Hands Behind.

(ix.) From Rest, Circle with Both Legs over Right Bar Right, with Half Right Turn to Half Lever.

§ 481. The following exercises are combinations of the vaults, leg circles, etc., hitherto described.

(i.) From Side Stand at Side of Bars, Front Vault Left In, Circle with Both Legs over Right Bar Right with Quarter Left Turn, to Rest on Left Bar with Legs over Right Bar, Squat over Near Bar to Ground, and Straddle Backwards over Near Bar to Ground, with a Half Right Turn.

(ii.) From Side Stand at Side of Bars, Rear Vault Right In, Swing Back, Circle with Left Leg over Left Bar Right, and, without replacing Left Hand, Circle with Left Leg over Right Bar Right, with Half Right Turn, at the Same Time Swinging Right Leg to the Right, to Momentary Half Lever, Swing Back, and Rear Vault over Both Bars to Ground in front of Right Hand with Half Left Turn.

(iii.) From Side Stand at Side of Bars, Grasp Near Bar with Combined Grasp, Right Hand Reversed, Circle with Both Legs over Both Bars Right, with Quarter Right Turn to Momentary Half Lever, Swing Back, and Rear Vault over Both Bars to Ground in front of Right Hand.

(iv.) From Side Stand at Side of Bars with Hands on Near Bar, Spring to Rest on Off Bar with Legs over Near Bar, Squat over Near Bar to Ground, Straddle over Near Bar to Free Front Lever, and Circle with Right Leg over Both Bars Right with Quarter Left Turn, to Riding Rest, Hands Behind, Close Legs, Pass Left Leg over Right, Backward Circle with Left Leg over Right Bar and Rear Vault over Both Bars to Ground in Front of Right Hand.

(v.) From Side Stand at Side of Bars, Rear Vault Right In, to Riding Rest, Hands Behind, Circle with Right Leg over Right Bar Left, with Quarter Right Turn to Rest on Right Bar with Left Leg over Left Bar, and Rear Vault Right over Both Bars to Ground.

(vi.) From Side Stand at Side of Bars with Combined Grasp of Near Bar, Right Hand Reversed, Circle with Both Legs over Both Bars Right with Half Right Turn, to Free Back Rest on Original Near Bar without Placing Left Hand on Original Off Bar, Circle with Both Legs Right over Present Off Bar, with Quarter Right Turn to Momentary Half Lever, Circle with Both Legs over Present Right Bar Left to Outside Rest behind Right Hand, and Flank Vault over Both Bars to Ground in Front of Right Hand. This is an exercise of extreme difficulty.

SWINGING EXERCISES FROM REST.

§ 482. It is advisable to practise straight arm swings, that is, swings in the straight arm rest, a good deal at first,

swinging the legs behind you as high as you can with a
hollow back, and forward as high as you can, bending at
the waist. There is a tendency to bend the knees at the
end of the backward swing, and at first you may do this
quite unconsciously. You may vary the swing by straddling
and closing the legs at either end of the swing or at both
ends. You should also practise swinging in the straight
arm rest with a hollow back throughout the movement.

§ 483. *Swing and Travel.* At either end of a straight
arm swing you may travel either forwards or backwards
with a jump from both hands made just before the end of
the swing. The backward swing with a backward travel is
the easiest of these movements, the forward swing and
backward travel the most difficult.

§ 484. *Swing to Handstand or Shoulderstand.* Swing, and
carry the legs backwards with a perfectly hollow back till
you come to the handstand or shoulderstand. If you intend
to reach the handstand with bent arms, or shoulderstand,
you must bend the arms as you swing, gradually, beginning
to bend them a little after the legs pass behind the hands,
so that the upper arms remain parallel to the body as the
legs swing up. The first of these movements to learn is
the swing to the double shoulderstand, rolling over if you
miss your balance, as described in § 385. When you are
completely at home in this movement you may try to reach
the bent arm handstand, spreading the arms and rolling
over if you overbalance. Then swing to handstands with
the arms less and less bent, always rolling over in the same
manner if you overbalance, and you will at last be able to
attempt the handstand with straight arms; in this way you
will learn to swing to a handstand with straight arms, without running any kind of risk.

§ 485. *Swing to Right Elbow Lever.* Swing, and carry

the legs over the right bar behind the right hand to a right
elbow lever. This is difficult at first, you must swing just
high enough but not too high. If you do not swing enough,
you will be unable to get the body over the elbow at all; if
you swing too high, you will not be able to keep the back
hollow when you reach the lever.

§ 486. You may do bent arm swings, that is, swings in a
bent arm rest, and, with bent arm swings, you may travel
just as with straight arm swings; the travels are a good
deal easier with a bent arm swing than with a straight arm
swing.

§ 487. *From the Rest, Swing Back and Front Pump.*
From the rest, swing back, then, exactly as you reach the
end of the swing, drop to the bent arm rest sharply, swing
forwards in the bent arm rest, and, just before you reach the
forward extremity of your swing, straighten the arms again.
You should begin to practise this exercise by swinging in
the bent arm rest, and endeavouring to straighten the arms
as you swing forward; at first you may strain your chest if
you try to drop to the bent arm rest in the manner described
above. When, however, you have acquired sufficient
strength in the bent arm swing, you should, in doing a
front pump after a swing backwards, swing almost to the·
handstand, and then drop to the bent arm position as
suddenly as possible. There is a tendency, which you must
avoid, to bend the arms slightly before you reach the
extremity of the backward swing.

§ 488. A front pump may be done from any position
which will allow you to swing forward; for example, from a
handstand, or shoulderstand, or a riding rest with the hands
in front. A front pump may be followed by a vault in
front of one hand or by a backward leg circle, and, after a
front pump, you may remain in a half lever.

§ 489. *From the Rest, Swing Forwards and Back Pump.*
From the rest swing forwards; when the legs have just
reached the forward extremity of their swing, drop to the
bent arm rest, swing back in that position and, just before
you reach the backward extremity of the swing, straighten
the arms again. You should begin to practise the back
pump in the same way as the front pump, that is, from the
bent arm swing.

§ 490. A back pump may be begun from any position in
which you have the legs in front. It may be followed by a
vault behind one hand or by a forward leg circle or forward
straddle. You may also do a back pump to a shoulderstand
or to a handstand with bent or straight arms.

§ 491. You may travel with a pump either forwards or
backwards at either extremity of either pump. Pumps and
travels, combined with straight arm swings and travels, give
a considerable variety of movements. You may specially
practise front pump and travel forwards to a half lever;
also back pump and travel either backwards or forwards to
a shoulderstand or handstand.

§ 492. The expressions " front pump " and " back pump "
are sometimes used to include dropping to the bent arm
rest, swinging in the bent arm rest and rising again to
straight arm rest, sometimes to mean dropping to the bent
arm rest and swinging in that rest only, sometimes to mean
swinging in the bent arm rest and rising to the straight arm
rest only.

EXERCISES BETWEEN REST AND HANG.

§ 493. *From Rest, Drop Back.* From the rest, swing
slightly backwards; as you begin to swing forwards again let
the body drop backwards with perfectly straight arms, at
the same time bending at the waist and raising the feet so

that the body passes between the bars and you come to a hang with inside grasp with the feet above the head and a little higher than the bars. The movement is exactly like a drop back from the rest on the horizontal bar (see § 281). As you drop back, you must shift the thumbs over the bars to join the fingers. The drop back is not an easy movement; success depends on keeping the arms perfectly straight and letting the shoulders come well forward. It is advisable to begin by practising a drop swing, first from a cross stand at the near end of bars, then from a cross stand between the bars; and then to practise the drop back from the rest at the near end of the bars before attempting it at the centre of the bars. The drop swing from a cross stand is, of course, just like the drop swing on a low bar from the stand described in § 282.

§ 494. *Short Upstart between Bars.* After a drop back, as you begin to swing back, you may do an upstart exactly as on a horizontal bar. This is not an easy movement at the centre of the bars, because, unless the arms are kept absolutely straight, you will be unable to get the shoulders through between the bars. Of course if the bars are considerably too wide for you there is not much difficulty about it, nor is it very difficult at the near end of the bars.

§ 495. *Long Underswing and Long Upstart between Bars.* From the rest a long underswing may be done between the bars just like the long underswing on the low bar described in § 280. This, however, is an exercise of the very greatest difficulty. You should, of course, swing well back and drop between the bars with perfectly straight arms; but I have never seen the long underswing accomplished in this manner. It is usually done by swinging back and then bending the arms with the elbows well turned in, and slipping through between the bars with bent arms and with the elbows in front of the body. A long underswing may be easily done from a cross stand between the bars or at the near end of the bars, in the same way as a long underswing on a low horizontal bar from the stand, as explained in § 280. You may, of course, do an upstart between the bars after a long underswing; the whole movement is called a long upstart.

§ 496. You may do an upstart between the bars to a half lever, never letting the feet sink between the bars at all after the drop back or long underswing is finished. This is a difficult movement but will repay practice, because, when you have learnt it, you will have acquired such control over your swing after the upstart, that you will be able to bring upstarts into combination with other movements with great ease. An upstart between the bars may obviously be followed by a backward swing or backward pump; it may also be followed by a backward leg circle, without pause, the leg circle being begun almost before the upstart is completed. Again, you may straddle the legs rather before the upstart is completed and come to a riding rest; or, at the near end of the bars, you may follow the upstart by a backward straddle to the ground, which is a very effective movement. Upstarts between the bars, followed by a backward swing and forward leg circle, are very pretty combinations.

§ 497. *From the Rest, Short Circle between Bars.* From the rest, proceed as if you meant to do a drop back; when the feet come above the head continue your swing, hollow the back very sharply and let go, turn completely over, passing the arms between the bars in front of you and catch the bars again, returning to the rest. This movement is very like a short circle on a horizontal bar; it is very difficult and a little dangerous at first. You may do the same movement from a cross stand between the bars, and from this position it is a little easier than from the rest.

UPPER ARM SWINGS, ETC.

§ 498. Upper arm swings, that is, swings in the upper arm rest, require a good deal of practice; at first you will find that these swings are somewhat painful, but, after a little practice, you will learn to do them without any dis-comfort. The secret is to keep the arms very rigid with the muscles braced, so that the arms do not slip along the bars at all. The following is the usual method of taking an upper arm swing. In the upper arm rest, take a slight swing, then swing the legs forward above the bars to the second position shown in Fig. 21, then hollow the back as nearly as you can, raising the hips as high above the bars as possible, and throw the legs forward, returning with a backward swing. The movement has a good deal the same character as that with which you take a swing on the horizontal bar.

§ 499. *From the Upper Arm Swing, Upper Arm Upstart.* Take a moderate swing on the upper arms, as you swing forwards raise the feet above the bars nearly to the second position shown in Fig. 21, but with the waist slightly less bent and the feet slightly further forward. Then, at the moment you begin to swing back again, make a sudden effort and rise from the upper arms to a straight arm swing. The movement has much the same character as an upstart on the bar, and is not very difficult. It is possible to do an upper arm upstart to the half lever; checking the back-ward swing the moment the upstart is done, so that the feet do not sink below the bars at all after the upstart. This movement is difficult; but it should be practised because it will give you great control over your swing after an upper arm upstart.

§ 500. *From the Upper Arm Swing, Back-Up.* Take as much swing as you can on the upper arms, and, just before you reach the backward extremity of your swing, rise from the upper arms to a straight arm rest with the legs behind you. Success in this movement depends almost entirely on getting sufficient swing.

§ 501. *From the Upper Arm Swing, Jerk Up.* Take a moderate swing on the upper arms ; as you swing forwards, and when the legs have just passed above the bars, hollow the back sharply and rise from the upper arms to a straight arm rest, immediately bending again at the waist. This movement may be done to a half lever without much difficulty.

§ 502. *From the Upper Arm Swing, Roll over Backwards to Double Shoulderstand.* This movement is just like that described in § 394, done quickly with a swing, you should bend as little at the waist as possible as you swing up, and hollow the back rather sharply when you let go with the hands.

§ 503. *From the Upper Arm Swing, Roll over Backwards to Handstand.* This is like the last exercise ; but you must take a good swing, and the moment you let go with the hands, hollow the back very sharply and you will spring clear of the bars from the shoulders, and come to the handstand without passing through a double shoulderstand. If this is done with a very good swing, and you hollow the back very sharply, you may in this way reach a handstand with straight arms; this is, however, extremely difficult.

§ 504. *From the Upper Arm Swing, Complete Roll Over Backwards.* Begin as in the exercise described in § 502 ; when you let go with the hands, do not place them on the bars behind you, but hold the arms straight out at right angles to the body, roll right round on the upper arms, and place the hands on the bars in front of the shoulders once more, and swing forwards on the upper arms again. This is an effective movement and not difficult. You should try to keep the back hollow almost all the time.

§ 505. *From the Upper Arm Swing, Swing Up to Shoulder-stand with Arms in Upper Arm Rest behind Shoulders.* Take as good a swing as you can in the upper arm rest; then, as you swing backwards, let the legs pass completely above the head; at the same time let go with the hands; pass the arms backwards outside the bars, and take hold of the bars behind the shoulders.

§ 506. *From the Upper Arm Swing, Complete Roll over Forwards.* Begin as in the exercise described in the last paragraph; but, when you let go with the hands, bring the arms only so far back that the arms are at right angles to the bars, then roll completely over on the upper arms and take hold of the bars once more in front of the shoulders, and swing backwards on the upper arms once more. This is a difficult movement, and requires a very good swing.

§ 507. *From the Upper Arm Swing Backwards, Long Underswing.* Take a moderate swing on the upper arms; when you reach the extremity of your backward swing, slip the arms over the bars to the inside, at the same time shifting the thumbs over the bars, and do a long under-swing.

§ 508. *From the Rest, Swing Forwards, Drop on to Upper Arms, and Upper Arm Swing Backwards.* From the rest, take a moderate swing, when the legs have passed the vertical position in the forward swing, let the body drop back, at the same time bending the arms slightly, and let the upper arms come in contact with the bars, so that you reach the second position shown in Fig. 21, then continue as described in § 498.

§ 509. *From the Rest, Swing Forwards, and Upper Arm Upstart.* Begin as in the exercise described in the last paragraph, but do not bend quite so much at the waist, and do not get the legs quite so far back; then do an upper arm upstart, as described in § 499.

§ 510. *From the Rest, Swing Forwards, and Roll over Backwards.* You may, after swinging forwards and dropping into the upper arms, as described in § 508, roll over backwards to the double shoulderstand, or to a handstand, or you may do a complete roll over backwards; you begin as in the exercise described in § 508, then continue as in the exercises described in §§ 502–504.

§ 511. *From the Rest, Swing Back, Drop on to Upper Arms, and Upper Arm Swing Forwards.* Swing backwards boldly, then, just before the legs have reached their highest point, let the shoulders move backwards, at the same time bending the arms very slightly, let the upper arms come in contact with the bars, and swing forwards on the upper arms. When the arms come in contact with the bars, the body and legs should be horizontal.

§ 512. You may drop to the upper arm swing from a shoulderstand or handstand, in a manner similar to that described in the last paragraph. Again, from a double shoulderstand, you may let go with both hands, pass the arms forward, take hold of the bars in front of the shoulders, and do an upper arm swing forwards.

§ 513. *From the Double Shoulderstand, Roll over, and Upper Arm Upstart.* The first part of this movement is exactly like that described in § 393, except that it should be done rather more quickly; then, as soon as you have got hold of the bars again, do an upper arm upstart.

§ 514. *From the Double Shoulderstand, Roll over, and Upper Arm Swing Backwards.* Roll over as in the exercise described in the last paragraph, but without bending at the waist, and swing back on the upper arms.

§ 515. The exercises described in §§ 498–514 are the most characteristic and effective movements on the parallel bars, and they lend themselves to extremely pretty combinations, with regard to which I may make some suggestions.

(i.) After an upper arm upstart, you may swing back to a handstand or shoulderstand, or swing back and do a forward straddle or leg circle; or you may, by checking the swing, follow the upper arm upstart, immediately, by a backward leg circle.

(ii.) You may follow a back-up from the upper arm swing by a vault behind the hands, or by a handstand or shoulderstand, or by a leg circle, or straddle, forwards. The back-up and shoulderstand, or handstand, is extremely difficult to do neatly.

(iii.) You may follow a jerk up with a vault in front of the hands, or by a leg circle backwards.

(iv.) You may do a roll over from the double shoulderstand, and do a back-up, proceeding as described in § 514.

(v.) You may do a roll over backwards to a handstand, and then drop on to the upper arms again, and repeat the movement or do a complete roll over backwards.

(vi.) You may obtain an upper arm swing from a cross stand at the near end of the bars, with a jump forwards; this is a very pretty way of beginning exercises.

SWINGING EXERCISES WITH TURNS.

§ 516. *Front Pump and Half Left Turn.* Do a front pump, and at the moment at which you would let go if you were doing a front pump and travel, let go and do a sharp half left turn in the air and catch the bars again. This turn should be done after as bold a pump as you can do, so that, during the turn, the legs are fairly above the bars, and you should catch the bars again with straight arms before the feet drop below the bars.

§ 517. A turn, similar to that described in the last paragraph, may be done after a forward swing with straight arms, or after a forward upper arm swing and a jerk up; but these turns, especially the first, are extremely difficult.

§ 518. *Front Pump and Shears with a Half Left Turn.* Begin as in the exercise described in § 516, but, as you turn, straddle the legs and alight on the bars in a riding rest with the hands in front. This is not a difficult movement to accomplish, but it is not at all easy to do well; you should let go both hands at once, do your turn fairly in the air, and let both hands and both legs come in contact with the bars simultaneously, alighting in a riding rest with the back quite hollow.

§ 519. Shears may be done after a forward swing with straight arms, or after a forward swing on the upper arms and a jerk up. These movements are difficult, but not so difficult as the turns described in § 517.

§ 520. A turn may be done after a back pump, but it is exceedingly difficult, and I have never seen it done myself. A similar turn might perhaps be done with a straight arm swing backwards.

§ 521. A back pump or backward swing and shears may be done. You should of course let go with both hands at once, turn in the air, and alight on the bars in a riding rest with hands behind; but I have never seen the movements done properly. The usual thing is to let the legs swing up behind, then turn the hips and straddle the legs, and then, when the legs come in contact with the bars, let go with the hands and turn the shoulders. Done like this, the movements are very ungainly.

MISCELLANEOUS EXERCISES.

§ 522. *Mounts from Cross Stand at Near End of Bars.*

(i.) From a cross stand at the near end of the bars you may do a back straddle mount to a riding seat on the bars in the same way as on the horse placed lengthways (see § 154).

(ii.) From the same position you may do a front vault right in, to a riding rest. Spring, and carry the legs over the right bar, at the same time shifting the right hand on to the left bar and doing a half left turn sharply, then straddle the legs, shift the left hand on to the original right bar, and alight in the riding rest ; you must endeavour to let both thighs come in contact with the bars simultaneously.

(iii.) From the same position, you may do a front vault right in to a momentary front lever in the rest. This movement is like that last described, but you must let go both hands at once and turn very sharply.

§ 523. From a handstand at the further end of the bars you may do an overthrow or high front vault, or a straddle to ground. These movements require no particular description.

§ 524. You may reach a handstand on one bar in various ways from a side position, and from such a handstand you may continue with various movements.

(i.) From the side stand at the side of the bars, you may spring to a handstand on the near bar.

(ii.) With a run, you may spring to a handstand on the off bar in a manner similar to that described in § 460.

(iii.) You may throw up to a handstand on the off bar from a rest on the off bar with legs over near bar.

(iv.) You may spring to a handstand on the off bar from a side stand between the bars, either straddling the legs or bending the knees to clear the near bar.

§ 525. From the handstand on the off bar you may do an overthrow, or squat, or straddle, to the ground; or you may let the legs sink to a rest on the off bar with the legs over the near bar; or you may turn to a handstand on both bars.

From the handstand on the near bar you may do an overthrow, or turn to a handstand on both bars, or step across to a handstand on the off bar.

§ 526. From a cross seat on the right bar with the left knee bent, and with the left hand on the left bar, you may do a vault or leg circle over both bars without touching the bars with the right hand.

§ 527. From the side stand at the side of the bars you may do a long upstart on the near bar, continuing with a vault in, or with some of the movements described in §§ 452–473. This upstart is difficult, because the off bar gets in the way; the feet must not come between the bars.

§ 528. You may do a long underswing on the near bar, and then pass the feet between the arms and do a half free seat circle forwards, either to a back rest on the near bar with the legs over the off bar, or to the ground beyond the off bar.

§ 529. From a side stand with the hands on the off bar, and the arms under the near bar, so that the near bar is more or less under your chin, you may do a short circle over the off bar and either come to the ground or to the rest on the off bar with legs over the near bar, or as you finish the short circle you may push off as if to come to the ground, but catch the near bar as you pass and continue with an upstart as described in § 527, or with the exercise described in the last paragraph.

§ 530. From the back rest on the off bar you may fall back and throw up to a momentary stand on the back of the neck, and then drop to the ground as described in § 409, making the whole movement quickly and hollowing the back sharply as you alight. This movement is called a " roll over backwards to the ground."

§ 531. The shear mount described in § 381 may be done quickly either from a side stand at side of the bars, or after dropping back from the rest on the near bar.

COMBINED EXERCISES.

§ 532. In this paragraph I shall give a few combined exercises, placing references in parentheses to the paragraphs where the movements introduced are described, wherever there seems to be any difficulty in the description. I may first point out that on the parallel bars slow exercises may be effectively combined with quick exercises, and also that effective combinations may be devised, finishing with exercises at the ends of the bars ; the latter combinations, however, must be arranged with reference to the length of the bars and to your own height, so that it is no use to give examples of such exercises.

(i.) From the Cross Stand at Near End of Bars, Forward Circle with Right Leg over Right Bar (§ 430), Swing Back, Forward Circle with Left Leg over Left Bar to Momentary Half Lever (§ 433), Straddle Legs to Riding Seat, Place Hands in Front, Close Legs, Swing Forward, and Rear Vault to Ground in Front of Right Hand (§ 421).

(ii.) From Side Stand at Side of Bars, Front Vault Left In (§ 475), Swing Forwards, Upper Arm Upstart (§ 509), Swing Back, Circle with Left Leg over Both Bars Right to

Rest with Left Leg over Right Bar in Front of Right Hand (§ 443), Swing Right Leg Back and Screw Circle with Right Leg over Both Bars Left with Half Left Turn to Riding Rest, Hands in Front (§ 480), Close Legs, Swing Forwards and Flank Vault in Front of Right Hand to Ground.

(iii.) From Cross Stand at Near End of Bars, Short Upstart, Backward Circle with Right Leg over Right Bar (§ 496), Forward Circle with Both Legs over Left Bar, Swing to Right Elbow Lever (§ 485), Let go with Left Hand, Replace Left Hand, Lift to Double Shoulderstand (§ 414), Roll over and Upper Arm Upstart (§ 513), Forward Pump and Travel, Backward Swing and Backward Travel to Double Shoulderstand, Roll over and Back-Up (§ 515), and Front Vault behind Right Hand to Ground.

(iv.) From Cross Stand at Near End of Bars, Jump to Upper Arm Swing at Centre of Bars, Complete Roll over Backwards (§ 504), Upper Arm Upstart to Handstand, Front Pump and Half Left Turn (§ 516), Forward Swing and Shears (§ 519), Place Hands Behind, Close Legs, Short Upstart Between Bars (§ 494), Forward Circle with Left Leg over Left Bar, and, without replacing Left Hand, Rear Vault in front of Right Hand to Ground.

(v.) From Side Stand at Side of Bars with Combined Grasp of Near Bar, Right Hand Reversed, Circle with Both Legs over Both Bars Right with Quarter Right Turn to Momentary Half Lever (§ 479), Swing to Handstand, Sink to Double Shoulderstand, Roll over, Back-up, Straddle Forwards, Back Pump with Backward Travel to Double Shoulderstand, Roll over, Swing Back on Upper Arms, Long Upstart Between Bars (§ 507), Circle with Both Legs over Right Bar Left with Quarter Left Turn to Rest on Left Bar with Legs over Right Bar and Straddle over Both Bars to Ground.

FRANK BRYAN,

38, CHARTERHOUSE SQUARE, LONDON, E.C.

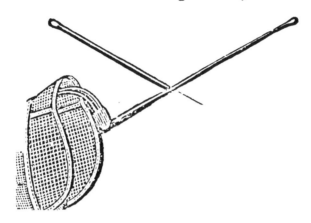

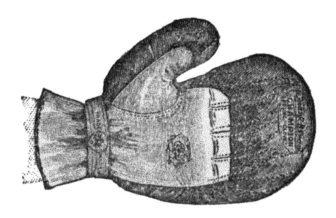

MANUFACTURER OF

FENCING GOODS, BOXING GLOVES,

INDIAN CLUBS, CALISTHENICS,

AND

GYMNASTIC APPARATUS, Etc.

PRICE LIST ON APPLICATION.

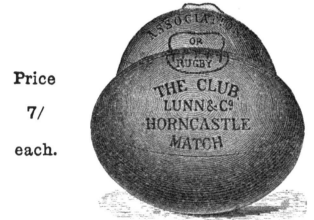

9 780260 845597